T0234507

Illuminating the Dark Side of Occupation

This innovative volume introduces Twinley's concept of 'The Dark Side of Occupation'. Focused on less explored and under-addressed occupations, it is an idea which challenges traditional assumptions around the positive, beneficial, health-promoting relationship between occupation and health.

Emphasising that people's individual experiences of occupations are not always addressed and may not always be legal, socially acceptable, or conducive to good health, the book investigates how these experiences can be explored theoretically, in practice and research, and in curriculum content for those learning about occupation. Beginning with a discussion of some assumptions and misunderstandings that have been made about the concept, the substantive chapters present and analyse tangible examples of the concept's applicability. This ground-breaking and practice-changing text provides ideas for future research and highlights contemporary, internationally relevant issues and concerns, such as the coronavirus pandemic.

This book is an essential purchase for students in occupational therapy and science, and valuable supplementary reading for practitioners. It is also relevant to a wide interdisciplinary audience with an interest in human occupation, encompassing anthropologists, councillors, criminologists, nurses, and human geographers.

Rebecca Twinley (known to many as 'Bex') recently took up the post of Senior Lecturer on the Occupational Therapy Programme at the University of Brighton. Bex is creator of the concept 'The Dark Side of Occupation', which has been attracting increasing global attention. Bex has been an approved member of the *Occupational Therapy Europe Register of Experts* in the area of dark side of occupation since May 2019. Her doctoral work focused on the lack of acknowledgement regarding a form of sexual offending that had been ignored: woman-to-woman rape and sexual assault. She enjoys thinking critically, challenging norms and assumptions, or just the plain and obvious lack of address of issues that impact upon people and their subjective experiences of occupations. Bex lives in East Sussex, UK and works at the University of Brighton, which she calls her "occupational home".

Routledge Advances in Occupational Science and Occupational Therapy

Occupational Therapy and Spirituality
Barbara Hemphill

Illuminating the Dark Side of Occupation
International Perspectives from Occupational Therapy and
Occupational Science
Rebecca Twinley

For more information about this series, please visit: www.routledge.com/
Routledge-Advances-in-Occupational-Science-and-Occupational-Therapy/book-
series/RAOSOT

Illuminating the Dark Side of Occupation

International Perspectives from Occupational Therapy and Occupational Science

Edited by Rebecca Twinley

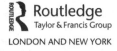

Routledge
Taylor & Francis Group

LONDON AND NEW YORK

First published 2021
by Routledge
2 Park Square, Milton Park, Abingdon, Oxon OX14 4RN

and by Routledge
52 Vanderbilt Avenue, New York, NY 10017

Routledge is an imprint of the Taylor & Francis Group, an informa business

© 2021 selection and editorial matter, Rebecca Twinley; individual chapters, the contributors

The right of Rebecca Twinley to be identified as the author of the editorial material, and of the authors for their individual chapters, has been asserted in accordance with sections 77 and 78 of the Copyright, Designs and Patents Act 1988.

British Library Cataloguing-in-Publication Data
A catalogue record for this book is available from the British Library

Library of Congress Cataloging-in-Publication Data
A catalog record has been requested for this book

ISBN: 978-0-367-21814-0 (hbk)
ISBN: 978-0-367-55776-8 (pbk)
ISBN: 978-0-429-26625-6 (ebk)

Typeset in Goudy
by Wearset Ltd, Boldon, Tyne and Wear

Dedicated to the loving memory of my non-biological mother, QC (Mel Joyner)

Contents

Figures

Tables

Boxes

Contributors

Editor

Rebecca Twinley Senior Lecturer in Occupational Therapy, School of Health Sciences, University of Brighton, UK.

Contributors

Kwaku Agyemang Occupational Therapist, Barnet Enfield and Haringey Mental Health NHS Trust, North London, UK.

Leonie Boland Alumni Research Fellow, University of Plymouth, UK.

Charles Christiansen Former Dean, School of Health Professions and Clinical Professor of Occupational Therapy, The University of Texas Medical Branch, Galveston, Texas, USA. Board Chair, Society for the Study of Occupation, USA.

Channine Clarke Principal Lecturer, School of Health Sciences and Academic Lead, University of Brighton, UK.

Mary Cowan Clinical Specialist Occupational Therapist and Team Leader in eating disorders, UK.

Miranda Cunningham Lecturer, Occupational Therapy, School of Health Professions, University of Plymouth, UK.

Amelia Di Tommaso Lecturer, Discipline of Occupational Therapy, School of Allied Health Sciences, Griffith University, Australia.

Priscilla Ennals Senior Manager, Research and Evaluations, Neami National, Preston, Victoria.

Roshan Galvaan Professor, Division of Occupational Therapy, School of Health and Rehabilitation Sciences, University of Cape Town, South Africa.

Craig Greber Assistant Professor in Occupational Therapy, Faculty of Health, University of Canberra, Australia.

Aliya Haddad (pseudonym) Palestine (confidential).

Claire Hart Principal Lecturer (Research and Innovation), School of Health and Social Care, Teesside University, UK.

Clare Hocking Professor of Occupational Science and Therapy, School of Clinical Sciences, Auckland University of Technology, New Zealand.

Karen Jacobs Program Director, Online Post-Professional OTD, Clinical Professor and Associate Dean for Digital Learning & Innovation, Boston University, USA.

Sarah Kantartzis Senior Lecturer in Occupational Therapy, Occupational Therapy and Arts Therapies Division, Queen Margaret University, Edinburgh, UK.

Kerrie Luck Postdoctoral Fellow, NaviCare/SoinsNavi, University of New Brunswick Saint John, Canada.

Carrie Anne Marshall Assistant Professor, Occupational Therapy, Western University, London, Ontario, Canada.

Elizabeth Anne McKay Associate Professor, Occupational Therapy, School of Health and Social Care, Edinburgh Napier University, UK.

Sarah Mercer Clinical Doctoral Research Fellow and Occupational Therapist, University of Southampton and Southern Health NHS Foundation Trust, UK.

Karen Morris Principal Lecturer in Rehabilitation, Institute of Health and Wellbeing, University of Cumbria, UK.

Julie Nastasi Assistant Professor, University of Scranton, Pennsylvania, USA.

Clement Nhunzvi Lecturer, Occupational Therapy, Department of Rehabilitation, College of Health Sciences, University of Zimbabwe, South Africa.

Jordan Pace Occupational Therapist, Dorset, UK.

Clarissa Sørlie Occupational Therapist, Step Up to Recovery, South London and Maudsley NHS Foundation Trust, London, UK.

S. Caroline Taylor Honorary Professor at Kwazulu Natal University, Melbourne, Victoria, Australia.

Quinn Tyminski Instructor, School of Medicine, Washington University in St. Louis, USA.

Lee Ann Westover EdD (student), Teachers College, Columbia University, New York, USA.

Gail Whiteford Strategic Professor/Conjoint Chair Allied Health and Community Wellbeing, Charles Sturt University, Australia.

Foreword

Out of the shadows – bringing light to darkness

It is useful to remember that occupational therapy emerged in the USA during an era in which societal attitudes and expectations were far more conformist and morally restrictive than they are now (Anderson & Reed, 2017). More importantly, those prevailing social norms dominated the contexts in which professional practice in occupational therapy and social work evolved. In his useful description of the evolution of social work, Reisch (1998) documents clearly that upholding morals and values was manifest in organised efforts to integrate and reform the impoverished immigrants and marginalised populations who were served by charitable organisations. These were exemplified by the settlement house movement (Christiansen & Haertl, 2018). What began as efforts to address urban social conditions and poverty resulting from immigration and industrialisation later shifted to a focus on individuals and their ignorance, character flaws, or psychological disturbances. For both social work and occupational therapy, the goal was to normalise the client into a productive routine of healthy self-sufficiency that was sustainable and socially acceptable; while also advancing the professional image of both enterprises.

Little wonder then, that for decades, the taxonomy of occupations advanced in the professional literature of occupational therapy was content to reside in the safety of non-controversial domains labelled as work, play, rest and self-care (Reed, 2005). During this time, the literature was nearly devoid of explicit references to activities that were potentially controversial. Consider human sexual occupations, for example. It wasn't just that mention of "sexual deviancy" was avoided, there was no acknowledgement that human sexual behaviour was even part of ordinary adult activity (Couldrick, 1998, 1999). And this avoidance extended to occupations seen as irrelevant or unimportant, such as sleep (Green, 2008), those that were illegal or undertaken as a consequence of limited opportunities, such as drug dealing or prostitution (Galvaan, 2012), or non-sanctioned, often linked to socially marginalised groups, such as hanging out, smoking, or gang membership (Kiepek et al., 2019).

Criticism of narrow, politically correct, Judeo-Christian understandings of occupation has included discussions of the dominance of white middle-class perspectives; thus reinforcing values and practices that marginalise alternative understandings (Beagan, 2015; Hammell, 2004, 2013). However, this marginalisation extends beyond non-dominant groups in the Western societies where occupational therapy was founded. The expansion of the profession around the world has led to the dominance of the English language across the professional discourse (Frank, 2012; Iwama, 2003; Laliberte Rudman et al., 2008), and the ongoing colonisation of local ways of knowing and doing (De Sousa Santos, 2015; Hammell, 2019). For example, in spite of our professed desire to respect cultural diversity, we have not engaged with how we can manage in one language a comprehensive discussion of concepts developed in another, and occupations uniquely named in a particular context and language remain in the shadows.

And even though many occupations such as sexual occupations and sleep finally became acknowledged as legitimate concerns within occupational therapy practice, it is striking that it has taken a century for the professional literature to begin to include a far-reaching examination of lifestyles and activities that have been socially marginalised or ignored. We wonder if this traditional reluctance to be more bold, expansive and inclusive in our thinking about occupation is a consequence of the profession's diffidence, its risk aversion secondary to professional ambition, or its lack of scientific rigour or imagination?

Understanding the occupational lives of those with whom occupational therapists work is influenced by our awareness of those occupations that are considered of interest or importance. It is inhibited by professional societies that acquiesce to societal demands for moral correctness or standardised efficiency, and also by the policies of the service environments within which practitioners work. In much of the 'Global North', constraints of budgets, reimbursement policies and biomedical understandings of health, within the broader political neo-liberal discourse, all shape the nature of services offered. For example, in both the United Kingdom and United States, therapists continue to focus on self-care in their practice with older adults despite the reality that social determinants, such as isolation and loneliness, are known to be of major significance to health (Ong et al., 2015).

These contradictions are also important because if occupational therapy is to be viewed as having expertise in human occupation for the purpose of enabling participation, our knowledge base cannot be influenced by convenience, tradition, or political correctness. We can lay claim to unique expertise in human occupation only if we command an authoritative and comprehensive knowledge of the topic, both specific to the person but also more broadly in terms of what is possible and what is valued in each context (Laliberte Rudman, 2010). Awareness of the cultural relativity of everyday life, of the tacit, situated nature of much that we do (Bourdieu & Wacquant, 1992; Giddens, 1991), and the limitations of our world views

(Gadamer, 1972), demands that we question what we think we know and how we can expand that knowledge to improve the health of individuals and populations.

We assert that a more complete, more critical discourse on occupations must be welcomed into the literature of research and practice. This will enable a full examination of marginalised, deviant, unhealthy or ignored occupations, their characteristics and relationships to occupational justice, and their connections to individual and cultural narratives as these reveal needs, situations, and lifestyles. Such an examination will surely enable both occupational science and occupational therapy to extend their understanding of the complexities of occupation and to reify a more authentic and inclusive vision of occupational science as articulated by Laliberte Rudman et al. (2008). We maintain that a complete and diverse understanding of human occupation, in all of its forms and contexts, is fundamental to ethically sound, socially just, and theoretically complete approaches to theory and practice (Mahoney & Kiraly-Alvarez, 2019). We congratulate Rebecca Twinley and her contributors to this volume for taking a major step in this direction.

Sarah Kantartzis, Edinburgh, UK
Charles Christiansen, Rochester, Minnesota, USA

References

Anderson, L.T., & Reed, K.L. (2017). *The history of occupational therapy: The first century*. Thorofare, NJ: Slack.

Beagan, B.L. (2015). Approaches to culture and diversity: A critical synthesis of occupational therapy literature. *Canadian Journal of Occupational Therapy*, 82(5), pp. 272–282. https://doi-org.libux.utmb.edu/10.1177/0008417414567530

Bourdieu, P., & Wacquant, L.J. (1992). *An invitation to reflexive sociology*. Cambridge: Polity Press.

Bushby, K., Chan, J., Druif, S., Ho, K., & Kinsella, E.A. (2015). Ethical tensions in occupational therapy practice: A scoping review. *British Journal of Occupational Therapy*, 78(4), pp. 212–221. https://doi.org/10.1177/0308022614564770

Christiansen, C., & Haertl, K. (2018). A contextual history of occupational therapy. In B. Schell & G. Gillen (Eds.), *Willard and Spackman's occupational therapy* (13th ed., pp. 11–41). Baltimore, MD: Wolters Kluwer.

Couldrick, L. (1998). Sexual issues within occupational therapy, part 1: Attitudes and practice. *British Journal of Occupational Therapy*, 61(12), pp. 538–544.

Couldrick, L. (1999). Sexual issues within occupational therapy, part 2: Implications for education and practice. *British Journal of Occupational Therapy*, 62(1), pp. 26–30.

De Sousa Santos, B. (2015). *Epistemologies of the South: Justice against epistemicide*. London: Routledge.

Frank, G. (2012). The 2010 Ruth Zemke lecture in occupational science occupational therapy/occupational science/occupational justice: Moral commitments and global assemblages. *Journal of Occupational Science*, 19(1), pp. 25–35. https://doi.org/10.1080/14427591.2011.607792

Gadamer, H.G. (1972). The science of the life-world. In *The later Husserl and the idea of phenomenology*. Dordrecht, Holland: Springer.

Galvaan, R. (2012). Occupational choice: The significance of socio-economic and political factors. In G.E. Whiteford & C. Hocking (Eds.), *Occupational science: Society, inclusion, participation* (pp. 152–162). Oxford: Wiley-Blackwell.

Giddens, A. (1991). *Modernity and self-identity. Self and society in the late modern age*. Cambridge: Polity Press.

Green, A. (2008). Sleep, occupation and the passage of time. *British Journal of Occupational Therapy, 71*(8), pp. 339–347. https://doi.org/10.1177/030802260807100808

Hammell, K.W. (2009). Sacred texts: A sceptical exploration of the assumptions underpinning theories of occupation. *Canadian Journal of Occupational Therapy, 76*(1), pp. 6–13. https://doi.org.libux.utmb.edu/10.1177/000841740907600105

Hammell, K.W. (2013). Occupation, well-being, and culture: Theory and cultural humility. *Canadian Journal of Occupational Therapy, 80*(4), pp. 224–234. https://doi-org.libux.utmb.edu/10.1177/0008417413500465

Hammell, K.W. (2019). Building globally relevant occupational therapy from the strength of our diversity. *World Federation of Occupational Therapists Bulletin, 75*(1), pp. 13–26. doi:10.1080/14473828.2018.1529480

Iwama, M. (2003). Toward culturally relevant epistemologies in occupational therapy. *American Journal of Occupational Therapy, 57*(5), pp. 582–588. https://doi.org/10.5014/ajot.57.5.582

Kiepek, N.C., Beagan, B., Laliberte Rudman, D., & Phelan, S. (2019). Silences around occupations framed as unhealthy, illegal, and deviant. *Journal of Occupational Science, 26*(3), pp. 341–353. https://doi.org/10.1080/14427591.2018.1499123

Laliberte Rudman, D. (2010). Occupational terminology – occupational possibilities. *Journal of Occupational Science, 17*(1), pp. 55–59. https://doi.org/10.1080/14427591.2010.9686673

Laliberte Rudman, D., Dennhardt, S., Fok, D., Huot, S., Molke, D., Park, A., & Zur, B. (2008). A vision for occupational science: Reflecting on our disciplinary culture. *Journal of Occupational Science, 15*(3), pp. 136–146. doi:10.1080/14427591.2008.9686623

Mahoney, W.J., & Kiraly-Alvarez, A.F. (2019). Challenging the status quo: Infusing non-Western ideas into occupational therapy education and practice. *The Open Journal of Occupational Therapy, 7*(3), pp. 1–10. https://doi.org/10.15453/2168-6408.1592

Ong, A.D., Uchino, B.N., & Wethington, E. (2015). Loneliness and health in older adults: A mini-review and synthesis. *Gerontology, 62*(4), pp. 443–449. doi:10.1159/000441651

Reed, K. (2005). An annotated history of the concepts in occupational therapy. In C. Christiansen, C.M. Baum, & J. Bass-Haugen (Eds.), *Occupational therapy: Performance, participation, and well-being* (pp. 567–628). Thorofare, NJ: Slack.

Reisch, M. (1998). The sociopolitical context and social work method, 1890–1950. *Social Service Review, 72*(2), pp. 161–181.

Preface

I had never really experienced writer's block until it came to writing this preface. I have opened almost every book on my shelves to search for examples of how other authors and editors have written a preface. My publisher's guidelines state: "A personal piece written by the author explaining how the book came to be written, or as a brief apologia" (Taylor & Francis, 2017). "Okay", I thought, "I can do personal – I work and write auto/biographically". But then I had to resort to Google: I typed in "apologia" and discovered it means "a formal written defence of one's opinions or conduct" (Oxford Dictionaries, 2019). So, I need to explain how this book came to be and to defend my opinions; I'll give it my best shot.

How this book came to be

In 2003 I took a career turn and started to train on a pre-registration MSc programme as an occupational therapist at the University of Brighton. The focus on occupation was so strong in this programme, yet it seemed to take me a while until I realised I did understand what occupation was, or could be. At the same time, I immediately questioned why the literature available to me at this time, and the evidence I was drawing upon to support and inform my learning, focused on promoting health (and wellbeing) through occupation. It really bothered, confused, and surprised me that so many other occupations were not written or spoken about. I could not understand this apparent omission in the theory that supports occupational therapy practice. I worried about how I would practise in what I was learning to be the ideal way – a way that is centred around and inclusive of the whole of (amongst other things) the person's interests, needs, concerns, skills, situations, capacities, and hopes. How would I achieve this if I only pay attention to occupations that have an obvious link to health and/or wellbeing? Those that are deemed socially acceptable or tolerated? Those that generally fall into categories that describe occupations as the daily, often routine, things people do? This concern and these questions stayed with me, through my time in practice, and it was when I started to work at a university that I found the headspace to be able to firm up my thoughts and relate them to the trickle of emerging literature I was seeking out that seemed to echo or hint at this gap in our underlying theory.

This book came to be. It came to be! But it did so after I travelled a long journey to get to this point – along the way I have encountered resistance to my ideas, misunderstandings, misrepresentations, judgements, assumptions, limited support, instances of disrespect, and, even, personal slander.

This book came to be because there were also some people who just "got it" and understood my concerns and intention. Thanks to the support of people who understand the intention behind this concept, this book constitutes the first collection of works based either on opinion, previous theory, experience, or research that explores the less explored and discusses that which has received limited or no attention. If I accomplish nothing else, the fact you are reading this means I managed to achieve, to whatever extent, what I set out to achieve: to illuminate the fact that there are so many occupations we are yet to understand and examine. Thus, the theory and evidence base regarding occupation needs to develop in order to challenge pervasive assumptions about the relationship between occupation, health, and wellbeing. We are members of a global community in which each and every one of us has a unique and subjective experience of occupation (even when we experience a global phenomenon such as the Coronavirus (Covid-19) pandemic) – let us recognise, address, and support this more fully and authentically.

Overview of the book

The key intention of this textbook is to recommend a shift in current theory, research, practice, and education regarding occupation. Categorically, occupation is the core concept of the occupational therapy profession and its philosophical foundations. There is vital consensus amongst occupational therapists and occupational scientists that occupation is complex and multidimensional; it is, therefore, frequently re-defined and debated. Importantly, this means that the understanding of what constitutes occupation is ever-evolving and responsive to innovative conceptual developments.

The format of this textbook is an edited collection of contributions that present an international perspective of the dark side of occupation, and how – as a theoretical concept – it is (and can be) translated into research, practice, and education. It is therefore relevant for any students, practitioners, educators, and researchers who understand that people are occupational beings and have the right to access and experience diverse occupations.

I encouraged contributors to write in first-person where appropriate; as an advocate of the sociological auto/biographical approach, I maintain it is important for us to "own" our work and to embrace our positionality and subjectivity. Plus, this means it is necessary to constantly interrogate the workings of power in all relationships – academically, educationally, therapeutically, professionally, and personally this is of importance.

I was fortunate to gather this collection from contributors around the globe. However, I would welcome the many other internationally and culturally diverse perspectives related to this concept – ones that equally need including and exposing in the developing sharing of knowledge. You will see I have invited contributions from a diverse selection of people, ranging from authors for whom this is their first publication to internationally renowned contributors from occupational therapy and occupational science. This was important to me, as Editor, because it reflects the scope, relevance, and – I would argue – timely, if not overdue, nature of considering, exploring, and discussing the dark side of occupation for everyone. Not "dark occupations".

Acknowledgements

A very appreciative and huge thanks to all the dedicated contributors to this book. Many of you know that I have found the journey to reach this point often somewhat challenging and, sometimes, lonely. However, you and other friends and colleagues have accompanied me, as our journeys have intersected at different points along the way, and in doing so you have contributed by lessening these feelings. I have so many people to be grateful for and thankful to, so the list that follows is in no way exhaustive, and there are some people in my life I would rather privately acknowledge.

Karen Jacobs – you had the belief to invite me to write a chapter about the dark side of occupation, which became part of the platform to gaining the contract for this book.

Claire Hart – your chat worked and, with thanks to my first Editor at Routledge – Carolina Attunes – as well as the editorial board and peer reviewers, I was given the go ahead. Thanks to my subsequent Editors for guiding me through the new process of producing a book. And for increasing my word count. Twice.

The Elizabeth Casson Trust – I extend gratitude for receiving funding to attend the SSO conference which had been assigned the theme "the darker side of occupations".

Brock Cook and Amelia Di Tommaso for your enduring support, encouragement, enthusiasm, and tolerance of late night/early morning messages.

Clare Hocking for becoming like a mentor to me.

Nedra Peter, Sarah Kantartzis, Paula Kramer, Gayle Letherby, Michelle Perryman-Fox, Rachel Rule, Matt Finch, Tendai Valentine Mutsvairo, Marnie Smith, Fiona Fraser, Rosi Raine, Tanja Križaj, and the many students who contact me for reminding me why I was doing this.

Dani Hitch for doing the work you do, being a guru, becoming a friend, and belonging in my go-to network of amazing people (see what I did there?!).

Geraldine Brown – your reflections were useful, thank you.

1 The dark side of occupation

An introduction to the naming, creation, development, and intent of the concept

Rebecca Twinley

Naming the concept: when a little bit of disruption navigates some change

I chose to begin this chapter with the issues that have been brought up through various forums (Twitter being the one I mostly use) regarding my use of the word "dark". This has been perceived, judged, and assumed to either be a moral judgement or, even, to hold negative racist or imperialist connotations. There has also been a great tendency for people to inaccurately use the term "dark occupations". That is not my concept, nor what I chose to name it. After the publication of someone's blog post titled "dark occupations" there were Twitter comments that it is a "slick and careless term that seems to have been creeping into the occupational therapy vocabulary"; I agreed by simply stating "#thedarksideofoccupation, not 'dark occupations'". Other comments have included that "it makes them sound bad" and that "occupations aren't dark". I find these interesting because they derive from drawing on adjectives of the word dark that can be found in the dictionary as being "sad" or "evil", which would mean prescribing an inherent "bad" or "negative" quality. That said, if we really think about all the occupations people do and might experience, one of my goals was to challenge the assumption that occupations are always "positive" and "good", and to emphasise how occupational science and occupational therapy have overlooked many occupations, including those that are perceived or judged to be bad, negative, upsetting, demoralising, and evil. As my friend and colleague, Danielle Hitch, once wrote in a message to me: "occupation ain't all sunshine and unicorns".

The quote that follows is taken from an email exchange with another friend and colleague:

> The association to race irks me. As a black person, being dark is not a negative thing and it should not be associated as such. To problematize dark in that respect perpetuates the prejudice.

She wrote this to me after I had shared some of the comments on Twitter with her, including one that stated "dark can be viewed as a micro aggression re race – ie dark and light". Personally, as someone who has experienced rape and interpersonal violence, this struck me because the term microaggression uses language that implies intended violence in order to describe verbal or written conduct. Further, White (2018) suggested "microaggressions are subtle snubs and slights directed toward minorities that are expressed unconsciously. But unconscious acts, by definition, are not intentional". So, if my use of the word "dark" has been received as a subtle snub or slight, or as crude prejudice toward you, I hope my clarification in this chapter diminishes such unintentional impacts. In Chapter 4, Hart suggests that, as a fledgling concept, the dark side of occupation is about the "unknown, unacknowledged, messy, and complex aspect of occupation", which offers some explanation as to why it can feel uncomfortable. Level of comfort is certainly a highly personal psychological state. For some, considering occupations that challenge the traditional assumptions made, especially those that focus on the links between health and occupation, can be challenging professionally more than personally. For others, personal views dominate and can cause a significant barrier to being able to consider occupations beyond the more traditional (which I would argue is mostly safe and comfortable) realm.

To be very clear for those who have misunderstood, I was not making a moral judgement, nor was I upholding racism – or shadeism or colourism for that matter – through use of the term dark. I am acutely aware that language is a potent force of our societies; for this reason, whenever I mention the concept I strive to be transparent: it is about occupations that have been hidden or not been implicit, and I would never suggest we should label other people's occupations as "dark" in any sense, as this truly would be making a value judgement about their subjective experience.

A terminological debate

In October 2019, Clare Hocking and I delivered a paper at the Society for the Study for Occupation: USA conference, titled "The 'Dark Side of Occupation': Creation and Intent of the Concept" (Twinley & Hocking, 2019). In this, we addressed the labelling of occupations as "dark" as opposed to those that are "in the dark". We spoke about how the former means that a moral judgement is being made about another person's subjective experience of occupations. Whereas, "the dark side of occupation" is figurative language pointing to the systematic lack of attention and exploration given to certain classes of occupations that have, therefore, been left in the dark. This terminological debate highlights the need to differentiate between viewing occupations as illegal/taboo/risky/unsanctioned (as the organisers of the conference had done), thereby stigmatising both the occupations and people who engage in them, versus the societal benefits of building knowledge of occupations about which little is currently understood, especially where there are real potential societal benefits of building such knowledge.

In our paper, Clare asked me: "On the topic of terminology, the term non-sanctioned occupation has more recently been proposed. How does that compare to what you're thinking about?" I explained that from my perspective, the work of Kiepek, Beagan, Rudman, and Phelan (2019) regarding silences around occupations and Gish, Kiepek, and Beagan's (2019) regarding substance use is exactly in line with illuminating less desirable, less known or explored occupations. I responded that I was aware Kiepek et al. (2019, p. 347) had labelled my concept "a pejorative framework" but that I felt we share the goal of trying to show the need for diversifying perspectives on human occupation. As I explained at this conference and in a more recent publication (Twinley & Castro de Jong, 2020, p. 24), my "intention was not to express contempt or disapproval regarding people's subjective experience/s of occupation; indeed, it was quite the opposite of this misunderstanding and misinterpretation".

On the topic of terminology, where I am based, in the UK, the term "sanctions" is predominantly understood in the formal sense. For instance, it can be the punishments levied on another country, or the penalties (in the form of benefits – or welfare – sanctions) imposed on people who are seen not to meet requirements for being a claimant of benefits from the government. Further, if we really consider language, sanction has opposite meanings – it can be an approval or a punishment. Hence, "whilst drug use might be sanctioned by law (and therefore made illegal), it might be sanctioned (as in approved of) or even promoted in the social group/s in which each individual person moves" (Twinley & Castro de Jong, 2020, p. 24).

For reasons such as these, I feel it is nether appropriate nor fitting to position an occupation along any kind of sanctioned/non-sanctioned continuum – especially because the very use of this language (or terminology) places normative limits, which I suggest can lead to a more positive/negative binary understanding of occupations. As a challenge to this terminological debate, Castro de Jong and I (2020, p. 24) felt that:

> sanctioned and nonsanctioned denotes that occupations either comply, or not, with social norms and formal or informal forces of control. By their very nature, occupations defy categorisation and are idiosyncratic; they cannot, therefore, be subject to binary interpretations. Understanding

occupations within context is crucial – influencing this consideration by introducing language that places restrictions on understanding is limiting.

Not a question of sides

The dark side of occupation is not another way in which to categorise occupations. Putting people, things, or occupations into categories is something we all do and is a process through which we are unconsciously biased – making judgements in order to make sense of the world. However, when it comes to occupations, we have the ability to challenge previous judgements and categorisations. To me, considering the dark side of occupation necessitates appreciating the absolute complexity and expanse of occupations: occupations which, therefore, present a challenge to the use of traditional and limiting categorisations which also have global inapplicability.

I am unique; you are unique. My subjective experience of occupation is just that – subjective and unique; so is yours. I cannot be put into a category; you cannot be put into a category. Why then should our occupations? Understandably, this can be useful in order to achieve focus or to offer accessible examples and descriptions in practice, or when students are learning about occupation. Nevertheless, with an increasing body of research about the array of occupations, our theory is evolving and so, therefore, should practice and education.

In 2013, I expressed how the fact that occupations are so complex means they cannot be separated into two sides, or neatly fitted into a certain category.

> Use of the term "dark side" is not intended to portray occupation as having two sides. As the definition and understanding of occupation has evolved, the great majority of accounts do now assert that occupation is something that is complex and multidimensional. It is certainly not something that can be divided into this side and that.
>
> (Twinley, 2013, p. 302)

Being human: subjectivity, emotions, affect, and critical consciousness

Just as a person subjectively perceives and understands occupations and the world, so do they when it comes to learning new facts, evidence, concepts, and theories. Social psychological theory has affirmed that emotions (as the observable presentation of how a person feels) and affect (as the non-conscious experience of intensity that facilitates people to feel their feelings) saturate our lives, shape our thinking and behaviour, and influence our social interactions and connections (Twinley, 2016; van Kleef, Cheshin, Fischer, & Schneider, 2016). How we feel about what we hear, or see, or read, learn, process, and experience is significantly influenced by emotion and our ever-changing emotional states (Tyng, Amin, Saad, & Malik, 2017).

In consideration of this, I have come to appreciate how the dark side of occupation is a concept which can and does have different meanings to different people; this is usually based upon factors such as their personal or professional experiences and interests, and it is always influenced by their own subjectivity, emotions, and affect as individuals and as unique human beings. I suggest it is necessary for each of us to be critically conscious, meaning that when striving for social and occupational justice, we engage in critical self-reflection. This does "not mean a singular focus on the self, but a stepping back to understand one's own assumptions, biases, and values, and a shifting of one's gaze from self to others and conditions of injustice in the world" (Kumagai & Lypson, 2009, p. 783).

By way of illustrating the differing ways people can respond to stimulus (in this case, in the form of a concept), I share some people's responses, expressed through the medium of art. First, an occupational therapist and artist called Susan Windeatt kindly granted me permission to present her artistic interpretation of my concept (Figure 1.1). As you can see, Susan

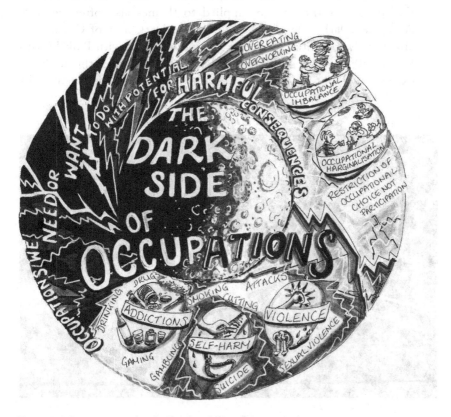

Figure 1.1 Interpreting the dark side of occupation.

Source: Susan Windeatt.

expressed her understanding of the dark side of occupation as the things people need, want, or perceive they have to do, and that have the potential for harmful consequences.

The second artistic expression (Figure 1.2) shared with me was by the creator of the Occupied Podcast, Brock Cook, and Occupational Therapist and contributor to this book, Clarissa Sørlie. In an email to me, Brock wrote to explain what their image represents to him:

> The Dark Side of Occupation has always drawn correlations for me with Pink Floyd's 1973 seminal album of a similar name. At the time Pink Floyd took a fairly standard arrangement of instruments and created with them a sound no one on earth had heard before. The concept album explored themes such as conflict, greed, death, and mental illness. Topics often ignored by songwriters before them. In parallel, the Dark Side of Occupation takes well-established ideas (e.g. occupation and Occupational Science) and highlights to therapists how they can be applied to themes also often ignored. And like "Dark Side of the Moon", The Dark Side of Occupation also has the potential to change the industry. As with Pink Floyd's famous album cover, this graphic depicts the variety of themes being extrapolated out through an "occupational lens", represented by the PEO.

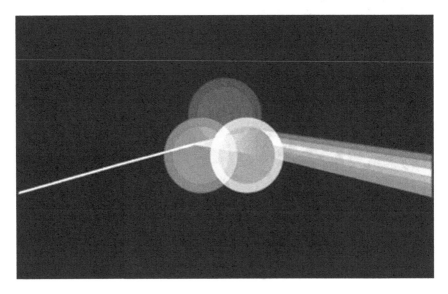

Figure 1.2 Interpreting the dark side of occupation.

Source: Brock Cook and Clarissa Sørlie.

Creating the concept

The image of the moon[1] used repeatedly in this text is deliberate: I am autistic and have a neurodivergent tendency to draw on visual metaphor to make sense of the world. When I was trying to make sense of the vast range and diversity of occupations, I imagined the dark side of the moon – the place where all those occupations are that remain out of the realms of our analyses, left in the dark, or in the shadows (Twinley, 2013) to our existing knowledge. To clarify, I was not romanticising through exotic construction. Indeed, aside from the use of the term "nonsanctioned", I concur with Kiepek et al. that:

> When examining occupations that are nonsanctioned, it is important to employ nonvoyeuristic approaches and avoid positioning the occupations and those who engage in them as exotic. Otherwise, we unintentionally reinforce the Othering of some occupations and some social groups, casting them as deviant.
>
> (2019, p. 349)

My concerns about a knowledge gap

All of this stemmed from when I was an occupational therapy student at the University of Brighton – a course that is deeply rooted in occupation and rightly so: occupation is the core concept of the occupational therapy profession and its philosophical foundations. As I learnt about health through occupation, I started to question why the literature I read only focused on health-giving or maintaining occupations. I reflected on my own lived experiences, and wondered why there was a very obvious neglect to consider the many things people do that take various forms, serve numerous functions, and can have a range of meanings; occupations that contribute to the formation of a person's identity and sense of self, that can provide a sense of wellbeing, or serve some purpose. The example I always draw upon is that at this time I was a cigarette smoker – something I enjoyed doing and something that helped me in social situations. Therefore, it was then that I began questioning why there was not a more nuanced understanding of occupations available for me and my peers to read and learn about. Without questioning these gaps, I felt I could not truly orient myself in the worlds of occupational therapy and occupational science because, very simply, I could not ignore the dark side of occupation.

Beginning to articulate the concept

In 2011, when I had been working in my first post at a university for less than a year, I realised I was increasingly uncomfortable with seeing students use definitions of occupation that excluded so many occupations, including those not perceived or experienced to be healthy, productive, prosocial, moral, or legal, for instance. At the same time, I was planning to conduct my doctoral research on woman-to-woman sexual victimisation; this meant I was reading a lot of work regarding violence and offending. Concomitantly, I was studying for a Post-Graduate Certificate in Academic Practice and met Gareth Addidle – a lecturer in criminology. We soon started talking about occupational therapy (he has previously been a nurse) and we decided to collaborate on a conference paper (Twinley & Addidle, 2011) and an opinion piece (Twinley & Addidle, 2012) to capture our combined opinion about occupations that are violent in nature – both of which marked the first instances where my concept "the dark side of occupation" was introduced. I was a new academic and this was only my second publishing venture. The paper attracted some critical appraisal that I had not been made aware of prior to its publication, but which made valid points, in particular that: "violence itself is not an occupation but, rather, an instrument of certain occupations, such as crime" (Aldrich & White, 2012, p. 527). I apologise for my flawed articulation and, as a reflective practitioner, see this as a key part of my journey to articulating the concept.

Development of the concept

The consensus amongst occupational therapists and occupational scientists that occupation is complex and multi-dimensional means that theory regarding occupation needs to evolve. Theories and concepts are dynamic; they develop in response to change, debate, and empirical evidence – the latter either affords or disproves their credibility. The dark side of occupation has seen significant growth and it is the development of evidence to support its credibility and relevance that is now required. Part II presents evidence from research that relates to the dark side of occupation, and which demonstrates the recognition of issues where research from an occupational perspective has been needed.

Occupational science for occupational therapy

In appreciation of the legacy occupational scientists have left through their works, my thoughts are very much in line with Hocking who, in 2009, asserted occupational science research and scholarship must continue to develop to fulfil the discipline's promise of generating knowledge of occupation itself. The historical focus upon the links between occupations, health, and wellbeing has dominated the discourse. However, references to occupations that challenge this are now emerging in the literature. As a challenge to the traditional assumptions, in 2017 I provided the following definition of the dark side of occupation for a core (US) text: "Occupations that remain unexplored – such as those that are health compromising, damaging, and deviant – and which therefore challenge the pervasive belief in a causal relationship between occupation and health" (Twinley, 2017, p. 29).

Occupational science endeavours have the potential to expose research directions that can benefit occupational therapy practice. As Iwama highlighted:

> Occupational science promises to inform us more about the nature of humans as occupational beings (Yerxa et al., 1989) and to inform occupational therapists (Yerxa, 1993b) about the profound core concept of their profession – something that other academic disciplines singularly have purportedly been unable to specifically and satisfactorily deliver.
>
> (2003, p. 583)

As I understand, the progression and development of our understanding of people as occupational beings demands that we engage in discussion and debate regarding occupations that have been left in the dark. Occupational science research could shed light on occupations previously unexplored, exploring their form, function, and meaning, and, on that basis, debate their contribution to health (of individuals and society). For instance, in more recent years, I have valued seeing the conversations that have sparked, with colleagues talking about mindful occupation (Goodman et al., 2019), stalking (Baker, 2019), intimacy and sexual practices (OT After Dark, 2019). The dark side of occupation is a big space – one which I find exciting to consider, but challenging to address. In Chapter 10, Greber discusses some of the practical reasons for this challenge, such as the need to address illegal, immoral or unhealthy occupations.

For its development, the very nature of the dark side of occupation means it cannot be a lone venture; I value collaborating globally with peers who have and will join me on this quest! As a big space, there are so many possible future directions and priority areas for consideration in education, practice, and research that will, in turn, be integrated into the developing theory of occupation. Something that none of us can now ignore is the occupational impact and implications that Coronavirus (Covid-19) – a truly global phenomenon – has caused. Alongside the need for this evolution are many other needs, such as for occupational scientists and occupational therapists to become socially responsible, to act on climate change, to challenge barriers in health, care, and education (such as culture, access, availability, and language) and the ever-increasing political tensions, to promote and advance equality, diversity, human and occupational rights, to strengthen as a global and diverse community, to be proud, to be resilient, to accept when change may be needed, to flourish, and to be kind in a world where there is much unkindness.

Clarifying the intent of the concept

As my WordPress site (Twinley, 2020) presents, and in an effort to be transparent, the following is to clarify the intent of the dark side of occupation.

It is about

- My use of a visual metaphor of the moon with a dark side to understand there is a dark side of occupation, as many occupations remain less "seen", understood, and under- or unexplored.
- My belief that advancing our understanding of the whole range of occupations people subjectively experience could contribute to the ability to work with individuals, groups, communities, and populations in an even more holistic and authentic way.
- Understanding occupation as complex and recognising the dynamic interactions between people, their environments, and their occupations.
- Encouraging less stigmatisation of participation in certain occupations.
- Looking beyond prescribing an initial judgement and being critically conscious.

My intention was to trigger consideration of hidden, less known, understood or under-explored occupations that are important, or hold meaning, or purpose, or are necessary for some reason. I see that this ranges from those which are perceived or experienced to be very mundane, customary, or ordinary, to the atypical, unique, and extraordinary. Whatever their form, the aim is that more occupations must be revealed and explored – immune from value or moral judgements and free from simplistic categorisation – in order to enhance the understanding of occupation and to gain a richer and more authentic understanding of people's experience.

It is not about

- Perceiving occupation as (rigidly) dichotomous in nature.
- Making assumptions.
- Putting boundaries on the things that people do.
- Othering, by viewing or treating an individual, a group of people, or an occupation as different in a bad, negative or deviant way.

Conclusion

Globally, the Coronavirus (Covid-19) pandemic caused a climate of much anxiety and, amongst other things, a dramatic and enforced change to people's routines; all of this gave rise to changing forms, functions, meanings, and experiences of an array of occupations. This saw an upsurge in focus on hospital and community-based occupational therapy services. Before this, occupational therapists were also already increasingly working in diverse settings that included shelters, prisons, and refugee, asylum, recovery, and drug and alcohol services. Across all settings and services, more and more, occupational therapists are being exposed to occupations, and are directly working with people whose occupations are unhealthy, harmful, boring, misperceived, or those that are even killing them; more often than not, this work is taking place within challenging environments that marginalise, disadvantage, disempower, and alienate people. This makes us responsible to equip ourselves – to be ready and prepared to work with the diversity of occupations, people, and settings that we do already and will do in the future.

Many occupations remain in the dark – yet to be explored, especially in terms of their form, function, and meaning. There are those that have shifted into the dark, and those that have shifted into the light; the implications of that for occupational science are related to the contribution we could make to society by explaining why people participate in the richly diverse range of occupations that they do.

As I see it, we all have a subjective experience of occupation and we all grapple with terms and language differently based on who we are, where we are from, where we have been, what we have experienced, who we have come into contact with, and what we do. The name for my concept has achieved the intended: it has triggered discussion (on social media, amongst teams and colleagues), it appears to have led to conferences being held with themes such as "The darker side of occupations: illegal, taboo, risky" (Twinley & Hocking, 2019); there have been calls for papers in line with the intent of the dark side of occupation (e.g. "Illuminating occupations at the heart of social problems", *Journal of Occupational Science*, and "Things people do: Toward a comprehensive understanding of human occupations", *Journal of Occupational Science*); and, of significant personal and professional achievement to me, it has led to this first book, which brings together a collection of works from people who all strive for an occupational perspective of occupations that are not intrinsically always or ever linked to health or wellbeing, or those that have been overlooked.

Note

1 Sincere thanks to Ponciano (from Pixabay) who granted me permission to use his image, which is free for commercial use, no attribution required. Retrieved from https://pixabay.com/photos/moon-sky-luna-lunar-universe-1527501/.

References

Aldrich, R.M., & White, N. (2012). Reconsidering violence: A response to Twinley and Addidle (2012) and Morris (2012). *British Journal of Occupational Therapy*, 75(11), pp. 527–529. https://doi.org/10.4276/030802212X13522194760057.

Baker, S. (2019). Stalking: A meaningful occupation? Retrieved from www.rcot.co. uk/annual-conference-2019-rcot2019.

Gish, A., Kiepek, N., & Beagan, B. (2019). Methamphetamine use among gay men: An interpretive review of a non-sanctioned occupation. *Journal of Occupational Science*. Advance online publication. doi:10.1080/14427591.2019.1643398.

Goodman, V., Wardrope, B., Myers, S., Cohen, S., McCorquodale, L., & Kinsella, E.A. (2019). Mindfulness and human occupation: A scoping review. *Scandinavian Journal of Occupational Therapy, 26*(3), pp. 157–170. doi:10.1080/11038128.2018.1483422.

Hocking, C. (2009). The challenge of occupation: Describing the things people do. *Journal of Occupational Science, 16*(3), pp. 140–150. doi:10.1080/14427591.2009.96 86655.

Iwama, M. (2003). Toward culturally relevant epistemologies in occupational therapy. *American Journal of Occupational Therapy, 57*(5), pp. 582–588. https://doi. org/10.5014/ajot.57.5.582.

Kiepek, N.C., Beagan, B., Laliberte Rudman, D., & Phelan, S. (2019). Silences around occupations framed as unhealthy, illegal, and deviant. *Journal of Occupational Science, 26*(3), pp. 341–353. doi:10.1080/14427591.2018.1499123.

Kumagai, A. & Lypson, M. (2009). Beyond cultural competence: Critical consciousness, social justice, and multicultural education. *Academic Medicine, 84*(6), pp. 782–787. doi:10.1097/ACM.0b013e3181a42398.

OT After Dark (2019). OT After Dark. Retrieved from https://otafterdark.com/.

Twinley, R. (2013). The dark side of occupation: A concept for consideration. *Australian Occupational Therapy Journal, 60*(4), pp. 301–303. doi:10.1111/ 1440-1630.12026.

Twinley, R. (2016). The perceived impacts of woman-to-woman rape and sexual assault, and the subsequent experience of disclosure, reaction, and support on victim/survivors' subjective experience of occupation (Doctoral dissertation, University of Plymouth, UK). Retrieved from https://pearl.plymouth.ac.uk/ handle/10026.1/6551.

Twinley, R. (2017). The dark side of occupation. In K. Jacobs & N. MacRae (Eds.), *Occupational therapy essentials for clinical competence* (3rd ed., pp. 29–36). Thorofare, NJ: Slack.

Twinley, R. (2020). The dark side of occupation: a concept created and being developed by Dr Rebecca Twinley. Retrieved from https://thedarksideofoccupation. wordpress.com/.

Twinley, R., & Addidle, G. (2011, September). Anti-social occupations: Considering the dark side of occupation. Paper presented at the International Occupational Science Conference: OTs Owning Occupation, Plymouth.

Twinley, R., & Addidle, G. (2012). Considering violence: The dark side of occupation. *British Journal of Occupational Therapy, 75*(4), pp. 202–204. doi:10.4276/0308 02212X13336366278257.

Twinley, R., & Castro de Jong, D. (2020). Commentary on: Sy, Bontje, Ohshima & Kiepek. Articulating the form, function, and meaning of drug using in the Philippines from the lens of morality and work ethics. *Journal of Occupational Science, 27*(1), pp. 22–25. doi:10.1080/14427591.2020.1733924.

Twinley, R., & Hocking, C. (2019). The "dark side of occupation": Creation and intent of the concept. *Proceedings of SSO: USA Annual Research Conference: The Darker Side of Occupations: Illegal, Taboo, Risky, 7*, 50–51. Retrieved from: www. sso-usa.org/assets/docs/proceedings_2019.pdf.

Tyng, C.M., Amin, H.U., Saad, M., & Malik, A.S. (2017). The influences of emotion on learning and memory. *Frontiers in Psychology*, 8, 1454. https://doi.org/10.3389/fpsyg.2017.01454.

van Kleef, G.A., Cheshin, A., Fischer, A.H., & Schneider, I.K. (2016). Editorial: The social nature of emotions. *Frontiers in Psychology*, 7. doi:10.3389/fpsyg.2016.00896.

White, L.T. (2018, 25 May). Microaggressions: A critique of the research. [Web log message]. Retrieved from www.psychologytoday.com/gb/blog/culture-conscious/201805/microaggressions-critique-the-research.

Part I

Theorising the dark side of occupation

2 The dark side of occupation

Accumulating insights from occupational science

Clare Hocking

Introduction

The founders of occupational science identified it as a basic science, the purpose of which is to generate scientific knowledge to inform the practice of occupational therapy; just as human anatomy and physiology inform medicine and psychology informs psychotherapy (Yerxa et al., 1990). Because occupation is both the "ends and means" of occupational therapy (McLaughlin Gray, 1998), that implies two kinds of knowledge. First, therapists need a thorough appreciation of the relationship of occupation and health and well-being, to ensure the identified health issue relates to occupation. Second, to support the use of occupation as a therapeutic medium, therapists need in-depth understandings of occupation itself. This second realm of knowledge is the focus of this chapter.

To use occupation therapeutically, knowledge about it needs to be comprehensive in scope and sufficiently detailed to have practical application. Clearly, as a relatively new research field, occupational scientists cannot yet credibly assert that the knowledge base is comprehensive. Nonetheless, 30 years after its emergence, it is timely to consider whether the discipline's accumulating knowledge illuminates important aspects of occupation and whether any identified gaps are problematic.

Previous critique of the field identified that occupational science research is skewed towards the occupations of "able-bodied white women and persons challenged by disability or disadvantage" (Pierce et al., 2010, p. 212) and, sociopolitically, presents an individualistic, middle-class, Western perspective (Hocking, 2012). While valid, those critiques focus on the human side of the person–occupation transaction, overlooking shortcomings in our knowledge of occupation – the things adults with disabilities, or middle-class, Western, able-bodied Caucasian women, or any other grouping of people actually do to ensure survival and occupy themselves.

Looking to occupations themselves, health and crime statistics internationally provide ample evidence that some of the things people do, especially those done repeatedly, can damage the person concerned, distress others, destroy property, and kill people and other forms of life. Human occupations also have capacity to undermine civil society, destroy ecosystems, and threaten the health of the planet (Hocking & Kroksmark, 2013). News bulletins also reveal people living in conflict zones or the aftermath of natural disasters, who risk their lives and their freedom by pursuing essential and meaningful occupations in hazardous situations. This is the dark side of occupation.

Not surprisingly, occupational therapists and scientists' unremittingly positive slant on occupations that are healthy and legal has been called out (Pierce, 2012; Twinley, 2013). There is now a trickle of literature reporting on the occupations that remain largely unexplored, such as those that compromise health, or are otherwise damaging, disrupted or deviant (Pierce, 2012; Twinley, 2017), where deviance refers to occupations that are negatively sanctioned, prohibited, or illegal (Kiepek, Beagan, Laliberte Rudman, & Phelan, 2019). Seeking a "more balanced, broader and inclusive appreciation of human occupation" (Twinley, 2013, p. 302) means attending to such occupations; studying their form, outcomes, what makes them meaningful, and the ideologies, sociopolitical discourses and circumstances that foster participation in such occupations (Aldrich & White, 2012).

Illuminating the dark side of occupation

Occupations with known health risks are being brought into the light, including smoking, albeit from the perspective of smoking cessation (Luck & Beagan, 2015, see also Chapter 7), skateboarding (Haines, Smith, & Baxter, 2010), and sustained playing of a musical instrument to the point of overuse injury (Guptill, 2012). Occupations that might be characterised as unhealthy and deviant include recreational methamphetamine use (Gish, Kiepek, & Beagan, 2019), addiction (Wasmuth, Brandon-Friedman, & Olesek, 2016), and binge drinking (Jennings & Cronin-Davis, 2016). Deviant occupations, from a law enforcement perspective, include begging and tagging, a form of graffiti. Begging carries the risk of being abused by members of the public and the musculoskeletal strain of being static and cold (Johansson, Fristedt, Boström, Björklund, & Wagman, 2019). Tagging involves scaling buildings and other structures to place a tag in a prominent position, with risks of falling, inadvertent inhalation of spray paint, and apprehension (Russell, 2008). There are now also studies of occupations that have been disrupted by political circumstances: growing olives in Palestine (Simaan, 2017) and the everyday occupations of long-term residents of an internal displacement camp in Uganda (McElroy, Muyinda, Atim,

Spittal, & Backman, 2012). Both of these hold explicit health risks. The olive growers face forcible eviction from their olive groves and confiscation of their land. Residents of the camps risked being killed, assaulted, maimed and raped, either within or outside the camp, along with the impact of despair over the loss of children; frustration, idleness and boredom due to loss of traditional roles (men); and poverty arising from forced removal from their land and assets.

Identity meanings on the dark side

Reading across this scant literature, five common features can be distinguished. First, many of the occupations have an associated identity that marks both its centrality and its normality in people's lives; a smoker, skateboarder, professional musician, addict, beggar, tagger. The exceptions are interesting. The binge drinker identified as a young man, marking his perception that drinking is a "quintessential part of British life; entrenched and embedded into its culture" (Jennings & Cronin-Davis, 2016, p. 248). To be a young man is to binge drink. Similarly, the young gay men interviewed about recreational meth use seemed to simply accept it as an aspect of being who they are (Gish et al., 2019). A hierarchy of identities was also sometimes evident, with research participants differentiating their identity at different times depending on their level of involvement (heavy user, supplier, smoker/ex-smoker), or differentiating themselves from others (smoking buddy, someone who periodically "grabs a [skate]board and stands around" (Haines et al., 2010, p. 242).

Where occupations had been disrupted by external circumstances, the identity meanings were quite different. For Palestinian olive growers, that identity expressed resistance to expropriation of the land, through signalling the land had owners and as a way of actively reclaiming land from the occupiers. However, it also expressed a more traditional identity as people with responsibilities for protecting the soil and tending the trees – "caring for the trees as their own children" (Simaan, 2017, p. 517). In contrast, the scale of the occupational disruption for people in the displacement camp was such that the researchers termed it a loss of identity for men, women and children alike.

Rewards on the dark side

Second, the occupations offer rewards as well as risks. The rewards derived from playing a musical instrument at a professional level are very personal, as captured in one participant's description of music being "my whole way of communicating" such that life would be "so empty without it" (Guptill, 2012, p. 264). Skateboarding delivered satisfaction from perfecting a trick and an intense feeling of freedom (Haines et al., 2010), while tagging generated excitement, a sense of belonging and invulnerability, status and fame. Tags were a vehicle to both personalise depersonalised spaces and express resistance to oppression, censorship and colonisation (Russell, 2008). Smoking could be a reward for completing another occupation, a break, five minutes to oneself (Luck & Beagan, 2015). Meth use brought increased energy and focus, enhanced performance and productivity, heightened sexual pleasure, adventurousness and sociality (Gish et al., 2019). As an occupation shared with other users, addiction could reinforce relationships (Wasmuth et al., 2016). The researchers of binge drinking noted the stories told were "full of vigour, enthusiasm and drive for what he was doing" (Jennings & Cronin-Davis, 2016, p. 249).

Begging, while experienced as shameful, did generate income that could be channelled to supporting one's family and educating one's children (Johansson et al., 2019). Despite the circumstances, growing olives in Palestine was described as a collective occupation that brought all the rewards of families working together, singing, sharing food, enjoying nature, having picnics and hosting guests, while the children played and explored (Simaan, 2017). Similarly, the productive occupations of the women in the camp ensured survival, bestowed the dignity of caring for others, and for some, generated sufficient income to pay school fees (McElroy et al., 2012).

Risk recognition

Third, participants in these occupations recognised the risks. For skate-boarders and taggers, the risk of physical injury seemed to heighten the thrill of participation (Haines et al., 2010; Russell, 2008). Risks associated with other occupations were managed, rationalised, or deflected. Injured musicians set timers to interrupt practice sessions that might otherwise go on too long and exacerbate injuries (Guptill, 2012). Smokers and those addicted to illicit drugs tried to address the risks by abstaining, and made repeated efforts to manage their intake or quit, including using medications such as nicotine replacements or suboxone. When they did manage to quit, many launched into a raft of health-promoting behaviours (Luck & Beagan, 2015). Recreational meth users self-restricted the dose, frequency and timing to minimise the impact on work, finances and relationships. They also used sterile needles, safer injection techniques and peer monitoring, sought out a reliable supplier, and otherwise maintained a healthy lifestyle (Gish et al., 2019). The binge drinker reasoned that he could avoid social censure by not becoming visibly intoxicated, and limit the long-term health consequences by reducing consumption in 10–15 years' time (Jennings & Cronin-Davis, 2016). Beggars took a break every few hours, to exercise, stretch, get a hot drink. They learnt to become invisible, to deflect aggressive responses, and sat on cardboard or clothing to insulate themselves from the cold ground (Johansson et al., 2019). Olive growers embraced international volunteers to help with the harvest, and more importantly, provide solidarity and delay interference from settlers and soldiers by being independent witnesses (Simaan, 2017). Men in the displacement camp learned not to venture out, as those caught tending gardens or animals were most at risk of brutal attacks (McElroy et al., 2012).

An alternative way of viewing participants' response to the array of risks they faced is that each of these occupations has parameters that people who engage in them endeavour to control, such as how long and how frequently they participate, with whom, and to whom their participation is visible. Participants can manage or at least be aware of the demands of their engagement, for example, the difficulty of the skateboarding trick or the musical piece they are practising, the dose of the drug they are taking, and the alternatives available to them, such as different modes of income rather than begging, and how accessible those options might be.

The intertwining of occupations

The fourth commonality is that these risky and deviant occupations are intertwined with other occupations. Skateboarding, and most likely tagging, stand in contrast to less novel and creative pursuits (Haines et al., 2010). The pain induced by playing music was relieved by taking a hot bath (Guptill, 2012). Smoking punctuated people's daily schedule, took their attention from social occupations, created the need to "sneak" a cigarette so as not to be seen, and affected everyday decisions such as how to arrange one's hair so that it did not smell of smoke (Luck & Beagan, 2015). Incapacitating hangovers from excess alcohol consumption could abort plans to do other things (Jennings & Cronin-Davis, 2016). Recreational meth use prolonged participation in dancing, partying with friends, and sexual activities, as well as enhancing productivity in occupations such as housework (Gish et al., 2019). Addiction to illicit drugs could escalate into supplying, or to the point of displacing almost everything else (Wasmuth et al., 2016). Begging, an occupation that was available when other income sources were not, also meant sleeping rough and a poor diet to curtail living costs (Johansson et al., 2019). As mentioned, olive growing was intermingled with picnicking, singing and hosting volunteers. Men in a displacement camp, robbed of their traditional occupations of raising crops and tending livestock, might abandon efforts to support their family and descend into drinking, playing cards, hanging out and watching videos. Without that support, some of the women's occupational load increased to include queueing for water, collecting distributions of food, and anything they could find to do to generate an income, such as brewing alcohol, petty trading, and making charcoal (McElroy et al., 2012).

Occupations that attract judgement

Fifth, and finally, each of these occupations, or pursuing them to the point of injury, attracts judgement and, in many cases, negative sanctions. Skateboarding can be dismissed as foolhardy sensation-seeking, with skaters derided for failing to wear protective helmets, kneepads, elbow pads, gloves, or blamed for being a cost to taxpayer-funded health systems. Professional musicians can be blamed for developing musculoskeletal injuries, on the assumption that injuries are caused by poor posture (Blanco-Piñeiro, Díaz-Pereira, & Martinez, 2017). Tagging is classed as vandalism, and heavily tagged locations are perceived to be unsafe, reducing both trade and property prices, casting taggers as a public nuisance (Russell, 2008). Aside from increasing social censure in many Western countries, smokers judged themselves as addicts and hid how much they smoked to avoid judgemental attitudes (Luck & Beagan, 2015). Use of illicit drugs is classed as a criminal activity in many jurisdictions, with addicts stigmatised as "immoral, weak-willed, or as having a character defect requiring punishment or incarceration" (Institute of Medicine, 1997). The recreational methamphetamine users who participated in the study discussed here might be doubly stigmatised for both their drug use and their sexual practices. Binge drinkers are characterised as noisily aggressive, antisocial, or victims of alcohol marketing and unscrupulous "up-selling" tactics targeting groups in bars and clubs (Social Issues Research Centre, 2019). Beggars are alternately framed as vulnerable or are marginalised, discriminated against (Johansson et al., 2019), and castigated as a threat to public order. When olive growers in rural areas plant and prune the trees and harvest the olives, they consider themselves the rightful owners of the land, yet in the eyes of settlers and the Israeli armed forces, their presence is perceived as provocative and warranting removal (Simaan, 2017). People trapped in displacement camps become economically destitute, and might quite correctly be considered to be robbed of opportunities to instil cultural values and practical skills in their children, and traumatised by prolonged deprivation (McElroy et al., 2012). Judging them as vulnerable, however, would be to rob them of self-respect.

Conclusion

In bringing this chapter to a close, two points are especially salient. First, while much remains to be learned about the dark side of occupations, the knowledge that is accumulating reveals that occupations considered within mainstream society to be damaging, disrupted, or deviant do indeed harm people: by being exposed to health risks or actual harm, through negative self-perception, and as the recipients of harmful attitudes or actions of others. Nonetheless, these occupations share the features of other occupations. Primarily, that they are replete with identity meanings, that people have reasons for engaging in them, and participating in them is in some way rewarding to the participants. As well, this analysis has brought to light important aspects of occupation that have not been widely considered. One aspect is that people who recognise risks associated with what they are doing also respond to those risks in some manner. That might be by welcoming, even seeking risk, or by rationalising their participation, by putting protective measures in place or, like the olive growers, accepting the risks as unavoidable if other benefits of participation are to be achieved. Another aspect is the degree to which occupations are intertwined, sometimes directly affecting the performance of those that follow. While obvious, this is an understudied perspective on occupation. In addition, the concept of occupations being socially sanctioned, whether as worthy or questionable things to do, was borne out, with participation judged accordingly. This is another aspect of occupation ripe for investigation, both the positive and negative sanctioning of people's valued occupations.

The second point worthy of consideration is the impact of labelling aspects of occupation that remain largely unexplored as a "dark side". Darkness is irrevocably associated, in the Western worldview, as negative, lesser, dangerous, unhappy, problematic, even taboo or evil. All these connotations are evident in common expressions: the dark days of war, dark passages in scripture, the dark knights. Certainly, some occupations have been systematically "left in the dark" because venturing there is challenging for researchers. Yet there are others that are merely out of view. The survival occupation of resource seeking, defined as the "range of activities focused on securing income supplements, goods, and services to meet basic survival needs" (Aldrich, Laliberte Rudman, & Dickie, 2017, p. 2), is an example of an occupation so hidden it had not previously been named in an occupational lexicon. Seeking to extend knowledge of such occupations is imperative if occupational therapists are to serve populations relegated to the economic margins of society by the prevailing political agendas. Equally, there is a need to better understand survival, forced, dirty, highly repetitive, "foreign" and low-status occupations. However, as well as these, occupational scientists are in the dark about heroic, communal, celebratory, and extraordinary occupations. Thus, rather than "peering into the darkness", I propose the need to reflect on the kinds of occupations that remain obscured, overlooked, or simply in the shadows, because, as a young science, none of our scholars and scientists have yet ventured in that direction.

References

Aldrich, R.M., Laliberte Rudman, D., & Dickie, V.A. (2017). Resource seeking as occupation: A critical and empirical exploration. *American Journal of Occupational Therapy, 71*(3), 7103260010p1-7103260010p9. doi:10.5014/ajot.2017.021782.

Aldrich, R.M., & White, N. (2012). Reconsidering violence: A response to Twinley and Addidle (2012) and Morris (2012). *British Journal of Occupational Therapy, 75*(11), 527–529. doi:10.4276/030802212X13522194760057.

Blanco-Piñeiro, P., Díaz-Pereira, P., & Martinez, A. (2017). Musicians, postural quality and musculoskeletal health: A literature review. *Journal of Bodywork and Movement Therapies, 21*(1), 157–172. doi:10.1016/j.jbmt.2016.06.018.

Gish, A., Kiepek, N., & Beagan, B. (2019). Methamphetamine use among gay men: An interpretive review of a non-sanctioned occupation. *Journal of Occupational Science*. Advance online publication. doi:10.1080/14427591.2019.1643398.

Guptill, C. (2012). Injured professional musicians and the complex relationship between occupation and health. *Journal of Occupational Science, 19*(3), 258–270. doi:10.1080/14427591.2012.670901.

Haines, C., Smith, T.M., & Baxter, M.F. (2010). Participation in the risk-taking occupation of skateboarding. *Journal of Occupational Science, 17*(4), 239–245. doi: 10.1080/14427591.2010.9686701.

Hocking, C. (2012). Occupations through the looking glass: Reflecting on occupational scientists' ontological assumptions. In G.E. Whiteford & C. Hocking (Eds.), *Occupational science: Society, inclusion, participation* (pp. 54–68). Oxford: Wiley-Blackwell.

Hocking, C., & Kroksmark, U. (2013). Sustainable occupational responses to climate change through lifestyle choices. *Scandinavian Journal of Occupational Therapy, 20*(2), 111–117. doi:10.3109/11038128.2012.725183.

Institute of Medicine (1997). *Dispelling the myths about addiction: Strategies to increase understanding and strengthen research*. Washington, DC: The National Academies Press.

Jennings, H., & Cronin-Davis, J. (2016). Investigating binge drinking using interpretive phenomenological analysis: Occupation for health or harm? *Journal of Occupational Science, 23*(2), 245–254. doi:10.1080/14427591.2015.1101387.

Johansson, A., Fristedt, S., Boström, M., Björklund, A., & Wagman, P. (2019). Occupational challenges and adaptations of vulnerable EU citizens from Romania begging in Sweden. *Journal of Occupational Science, 26*(2), 200–210. doi:10.1080/14 427591.2018.1557071.

Kiepek, N., Beagan, B., Laliberte Rudman, D., & Phelan, S. (2019). Silences around occupations framed as unhealthy, illegal, and deviant. *Journal of Occupational Science, 26*(3), 341–353. doi:10.1080/14427591.2018.1499123.

Luck, K., & Beagan, B. (2015). Occupational transition of smoking cessation in women: "You're restructuring your whole life". *Journal of Occupational Science, 22*(2), 183–196. doi:10.1080/14427591.2014.887418.

McElroy, T., Muyinda, H., Atim, S., Spittal, P., & Backman, C. (2012). War, displacement and productive occupations in Northern Uganda. *Journal of Occupational Science, 19*(3), 198–212. doi:10.1080/14427591.2011.614681.

McLaughlin Gray, J. (1998). Putting occupation into practice: Occupation as ends, occupation as means. *American Journal of Occupational Therapy, 52*, 354–364. doi:10.5014/ajot.52.5.354.

Pierce, D. (2012). Ruth Zemke Lecture in Occupational Science: Promise. *Journal of Occupational Science, 19*(4), 298–311. doi:10.1080/14427591.2012.667778.

Pierce, D., Atler, J., Baltisberger, E., Fehringer, E., Hunter, E., Malkawi, S., & Parr, T. (2010). Occupational science: A data-based American perspective. *Journal of Occupational Science, 17*(4), 204–215. doi:10.1080/14427591.2010.9686697.

Russell, E. (2008). Writing on the wall: The form, function and meaning of tagging. *Journal of Occupational Science, 15*(2), 87–97. doi:10.1080/14427591.2008.9686614.

Simaan, J. (2017). Olive growing in Palestine: A decolonial ethnographic study of collective daily-forms-of-resistance. *Journal of Occupational Science, 24*(4), 510–523. doi:10.1080/14427591.2017.1378119.

Social Issues Research Centre (2019). Binge drinking. Retrieved from www.sirc.org/publik/binge_drinking.shtml.

Twinley, R. (2013). The dark side of occupation: A concept for consideration. *Australia Occupational Therapy Journal, 60,* 301–303.

Twinley, R. (2017). The dark side of occupation. In K. Jacobs & N. MacRae (Eds.), *Occupational therapy essentials for clinical competence* (3rd ed., pp. 29–36). Thorofare, NJ: Slack.

Wasmuth, S., Brandon-Friedman, R.A., & Olesek, K. (2016). A grounded theory of veterans' experiences of addiction-as-occupation. *Journal of Occupational Science, 23*(1), 128–141. doi:10.1080/14427591.2015.1070782.

Yerxa, E.J., Clark, F., Frank, G., Jackson, J., Parham, D., Pierce, D., ... Zemke, R. (1990). An introduction to occupational science, a foundation for occupational therapy in the 21st century. *Occupational Therapy in Health Care, 6*(4), 1–17. doi:10.1080/J003v06n04_04.

3 The dark side of occupation
A historical review of occupational therapy

Elizabeth Anne McKay

Introduction

As the great comedian Spike Milligan (2018) wrote, "Occupational Therapy twixt birth and death"; we are what we do throughout our life and what we do sometimes is not what we or indeed others would approve of – this includes those of us who may individually have negative thoughts or indeed actions. As a healthcare profession, occupational therapists have not, until recently, taken the time to consider those occupations that may not be promoting or maintaining people's health. This includes a range from those that are dull to those that are antisocial, illegal, taboo, or risky. Our work – whether practice, research, or education – has not been focused on what are considered "in the dark": here I will discuss why this may have arisen and what has changed. Twinley's (2017, p. 29) definition is useful here to centre our focus: "Occupations that remain unexplored – such as those that are health compromising, damaging and deviant – and which therefore challenge the pervasive belief in the causal relationship between occupation and health".

Personally, I have difficulty thinking about the "dark" without first heading off to the ground-breaking Pink Floyd album "The Dark Side of the Moon". Why you may ask? Well, until very recently the "dark side" was the undiscovered, unknown, and unexplored. However, now we have the technology, this is no longer the case, and we now know that the dark side of the moon is – surprisingly – much like the side we were used to seeing; indeed now that we can see it, there is little difference – the perhaps imagined things that could be in the dark were not present. So by throwing light, illuminating the dark aspects of engaging in occupations, this book may in the forthcoming chapters show many similarities, not differences. Back to my task: occupational therapy development and the dark side of occupation.

Whose productive occupation?

To start off, I am going to ask you to consider some aspects of our profession perhaps not known, not discussed, or not experienced by all. For example, as a student on my first placement in a psychiatric hospital in Scotland, I was encouraged to see that the long-term patients (I'm using this phrase deliberately), who were attending the day unit, were engaged in what looked like to me, a first year student, a positive and productive occupation of knitting. The patients worked hard knitting throughout the day and produced a good amount of knitting – so I was appalled to discover that at the end of the day their knitting was stripped back, and the next day they would start again: repeating the whole process again. While nothing about this shouts illegal, deviant, or risky, it should make us think about why therapists would organise this task? Was it promoting health? Or was it compromising their health? I believe it does say something about how we valued these individuals, how we did not offer them choice and limited their occupational engagement over a period of time; and I'm sure you can think of examples you have witnessed.

Another example of the profession sustaining meaningless occupations (which I use to refer to occupations that have no meaning, significance, purpose, or reason) for those involved is drawn from Britain, in the middle of the twentieth century. At this time people who were considered mentally ill or who had a learning disability often worked in organisations; where attendees filled envelopes, packed medical sticks, or sorted paper for days on end: intended to be "productive" for whom? The individual or the organisation? These people were fulfilling contracts normally undertaken by NHS of Local Authority organisations. This was considered to be therapeutic work – with the prevailing belief that work is therapy. Importantly, people had little or no say in their engagement, or in how meaningful the activities were to them.

This highlights the issues inherent when assumptions are made regarding what is deemed to be "therapeutic" or "meaningful" or productive. We can always acknowledge this was a different time and we, as a profession, were not as theoretically sophisticated as we are today. Nevertheless, assumptions are still made; perhaps because even now "theories of occupation are culturally specific, class-bound, ableist, and lacking in supportive evidence" (Hammell, 2009, p. 107).

Again we have to think about the issue of productivity – whose productivity? A less well known aspect of our history is how the profession in Germany was involved before the outbreak of the Second World War in the assessment of people who were considered "unworthy of life". Cooper, in her paper "Radical exclusion: Nazi euthanasia, 1939–1945", discusses "how productivity became a criteria for deciding which patients to include in the euthanasia programme" (2005, p. 22). Productivity as a sign of health and worth created an environment in which those who were unwell or unable to work were considered "incurable" and could be assessed by "occupational therapists" for sterilisation and later assigned to "work" camps. The past can be an uncomfortable place to look back on and these examples illustrate that we as a profession are not immune to darker practices.

A brief history of occupational therapy

The following section gives a brief overview of the development of occupational therapy, first in mental health, where I consider the growth of occupational therapy and its unique relationship with the early development of psychiatry (McKay, 2008). Throughout, the fundamental principle was that engagement in meaningful occupations was of benefit to the individual – a principle that occupational therapy was founded and expanded on later. Busfield asserts that "value was placed on reason, and unreason in all its forms – madness, crime and poverty was banished in a great confinement" (1996, p. 70). If we look closer at Busfield's words, madness (deviant), crime (illegal) and poverty were removed from society, indeed out of sight out of mind. This was undeniably a dark time; an unenlightened time.

During the eighteenth century – the age of enlightenment – the growth of moral treatment drew on the humanistic principles that proposed that "all men were made equal and governed by universal laws" (Kielhofner, 1983, p. 11). There was an emphasis on the humanity of individuals and the importance of the arts to humanity. Conceived by Pinel, moral treatment led him to introduce work to the Bicetre Asylum for the Insane, in Paris. He further prescribed physical activity and manual work, with the aim of reducing the use of external physical coercion. His reforms were widely recognised and followed across Europe and North America (Paterson, 1997). In the UK, William and Samuel Tuke, Quakers, founded and developed the York Retreat, based on moral treatment. They believed that by treating patients as rational individuals, they could be re-educated by structuring the environment physically, socially, and temporally; a programme of organised occupations that minimised disorganised behaviour of the mentally ill. Occupation as therapy was created – the forerunner of occupational therapy (Wilcock, 2001).

The early proponents of moral treatment in the USA were psychiatrists; all played a major role in the formation of the profession of occupational therapy. Rush was the first to use the concepts of moral treatment and occupation. Meyer reiterated the importance of occupation and treatment. His work had a significant impact on the development of the philosophy of occupational therapy in the USA (Meyer, 1997). It was Meyer who employed Eleanor Clarke Slagle as the director of occupational therapy at his hospital, and she established the first professional school for occupational therapists in Chicago, in 1915.

At the start of the twentieth century, moral treatment could not be sustained, with the result that most asylums provided only custodial care (Paterson, 1997). Nonetheless, work activities were still used with patients, but more for the maintenance of the institution rather than for the benefit of those who were mentally ill. Few establishments held true to the value of occupation both for the individual's own productivity and for their personal satisfaction (Jackson, 1993). Another thread which informed our early development was the "Arts and Crafts" movement which developed from the 1840s onwards; this movement rallied against mass production and its dehumanising impact on workers and communities. It focused on craft as a way to bring back integrity, both to the maker and the object. The new profession of occupational therapy working in mental health settings in the UK, USA, and Canada shared the Western belief in the efficacy of meaningful occupation as useful, productive, and health-promoting for the individual.

However, it was the First World War that saw occupational therapy develop into a profession that worked with those returning from the military front. This saw rehabilitation centres to treat physically and mentally injured soldiers, through the use of occupation that was predominantly work-focused – getting people back to employment; to be productive, to contribute to society was deemed important. This was particularly key against a background in which Europe had witnessed great turmoil, resulting in wholescale overthrowing of long-established regimes; for example, the fall of Russia and the growth of Communism; stable employment reduced the likelihood of greater unrest.

After the Second World War, in 1948, occupational therapy in the UK became part of the newly established National Health Service; occupational therapy provision was centred on the individual's self-care and work. It was predominantly hospital-based and focused on rehabilitation from mental and physical illness, such as polio and TB. Although, community services were beginning to develop through the 1960s to support people to remain at home or return home. Funding moved to local government authorities with a growth in community, or social care, provision; practice strengthened around self-care and work.

The 1960s and 1970s saw the influence of a range of theories and modalities impacting occupational therapy in mental health and physical practice: analytical psychotherapy, behaviourism and cognitive theories (Kielhofner, 1983). The profession was perceived as being in a time of crisis. The integration of such theories led to the loss of professional confidence and commitment to use of occupation. Reitz (1992) found that occupational therapy abandoned its earlier philosophy of occupation and health. Therapists had lost their appreciation of the importance of occupation and its significance to human life (Kielhofner, 1983; Whiteford, 2000). Since the 1990s, a growth area for occupational therapy has been within secure hospital settings, with the development of forensic occupational therapy services within the specialist State Mental Hospitals: specifically, working with people with a mental illness involved in illegal occupations (Duncan et al., 2003). In the past 15 years, there has been a slow growth of occupational therapists working in the prison system, working with people who were engaged in illegal activities.

What drove the changes?

I propose that it was a combination of various factors that emerged through the 1980s – including the move to degree-level education, increase in research, theoretical developments, especially the development of practice models, occupational science, and a greater diversity of voices – that enabled occupational therapy as a profession to begin to extend its vision to include the dark side of occupations. This was not a linear process, rather a pattern of different aspects impacting around the world.

The first of these key developments was the upgrading of the profession to degree programmes which encapsulated evidence-based practice and research methods. The profession took a leap forward in understanding the need for research that influenced and impacted on occupational therapy practice, leading to an uptake of postgraduate programmes and further upskilling of practitioners. This promoted different research within the profession designed and led by occupational therapists, with new areas and concepts being explored, tested, and developed. Moreover, the resulting need for doctoral qualifications within higher education facilitated a greater emphasis on occupation as something to be researched; importantly, from an occupational perspective, not only through a health lens.

Second, the refocus on humans as occupational beings, with occupation, occupational identity, and performance being identified as core concepts of the profession, led to the development of practice models: for example, Reed and Sanderson (1980), Model of Human Occupation (Kielhofner, 1985) and the Canadian Model of Occupational Performance CMOP (CAOT, 1997), and later CMOP-Engagement (in Townsend & Polatajko, 2007). These models shaped practice and served to strengthen occupational therapists' beliefs in their profession, and in the health-giving benefits of occupation. Practice evolves, largely in response to theoretical developments, as Kemmis (2009, p. 20) states: "practice is an evolving social form which is reflexively restructured and transformed over time". Moreover, these models enabled most occupational therapists to articulate the complexity of their practice, and the significance of the person–environment–occupation relationship; shifting from solely focusing on individual health to include engagement, context and communities.

The third, and potentially the most significant, driver of change is attributed to occupational science. This encouraged the profession to examine occupation as an aspect of human behaviour, something done in time with myriad factors impacting: not just illness and illness consequences. Occupational science developed as an academic discipline to generate knowledge about the form, function, and meaning of all human occupations (Zemke & Clarke, 1996). As a multi-professional discipline, initially developed at the University of Southern California, it built on the work of Meyer, Riley, Ayres and others, and the ideas put forward have generated worldwide interest and research (Yerxa et al., 1990).

It is argued that occupational therapy's unique contribution to health lies in the relationship between health and occupation (Wilcock, 1998), with Wilcock (1993) proposing that there is a human biological need for occupation. Wilcock (1998) stressed that the profession has negated the potential of occupation to influence the public health agenda. Occupational science theory has offered occupational therapists new ways of thinking and researching new concepts to broaden and sharpen the profession's horizon (Wilcock, 2001). It proposes that individuals should be studied in their interactions with their occupations and environment in everyday situations (Yerxa et al., 1990). "Occupation" is what people want, need, or have to do, e.g. physical, mental, social, sexual, political, or spiritual activities, including sleep/rest (Wilcock & Townsend, 2014). "Doing, being, becoming, and belonging" are central aspects highlighting occupation as a biological need for survival, with engagement in prosocial as well as antisocial occupations, which fill people's days (Wilcock & Hocking, 2015).

Core concepts of occupational science are occupational justice and injustice. Occupational injustice refers to situations beyond the control of individuals, groups, or communities that inhibit participation in meaningful occupations conducive to health and wellbeing, and this can prevail in various ways (Townsend & Wilcock, 2004). "Occupational deprivation" is defined as "a state of prolonged preclusion from engagement in occupations of necessity and/or meaning due to factors that stand outside the control of the individual" (Whiteford, 2003, p. 222). "Occupational marginalisation" is the inhibition of the right to exercise autonomous choices regarding participation in occupations (Townsend & Wilcock, 2004). "Occupational imbalance" is being over- or under-occupied, specifically related to the privilege of participation in diverse occupations. "Occupational alienation" is when individuals or communities participate in occupations that are not perceived as meaningful, enriching, or fulfilling to them (Townsend & Wilcock, 2004).

Occupational injustice in all its forms may be experienced by those engaging in occupations that are taboo, risky, or illegal. The examination of these people's experiences requires a variety of research methods that enable the illumination of our understanding of how people ascribe meaning to occupation and their lives, and how they experience participation or exclusion. Methods to achieve these aims have focused on using diverse methodological approaches, including qualitative designs such as narrative inquiry, Interpretative Phenomenology Analysis, and Participatory Action Research and methods such as Photovoice to access and present unique accounts (Bacon, McKay, & Reynolds, 2020; Frank, 1996; Polkinghorne, 1995). These methods are consistent with the central tenets of post-modernism, with its emphasis on different perspectives, situatedness, temporality, difference and contexts.

The rise of the Global South, including Latin America, Asia, and Africa, added diverse voices to the profession. Some of these different perspectives were captured in the seminal text *Occupational Therapy without borders: Learning from the spirit of survivors* (Kronenberg, Algado, & Pollard, 2001); it introduced occupational apartheid and presented different world perspectives to the wider world. Furthermore, the deliberate strategy by the World Federation of Occupational Therapists (WFOT) to engage with the Global South has enabled practitioners and researchers to showcase their distinct practice through WFOT conferences: Chile, 2010, Japan, 2014, and most recently South Africa, 2018. As people have examined these global perspectives in depth, occupational therapy, in the process, has been repositioned beyond its traditional health and social care borders to examine wider society, social justice, inclusion, and those living in the margins or engaged in the dark side of occupation.

To conclude, as we move forward we need to understand how our historical roots and recent past have shaped our development in practice, research, and education. As Hocking explores in Chapter 2, there is growing theoretical and research literature concerning occupational justice and injustice, with some illuminating the dark side of occupations, such as those that are violent (Twinley & Addidle, 2012); substance abuse (Bacon et al., 2020); addiction and impulse control disorders (Kiepek & Magalhães, 2011); and considering race and racism (Nicholls & Elliot, 2018). All aim to expand our vision and thinking, and to promote the need to research unexplored occupations of diverse populations. Occupational therapy needs to respond and look into the dark side of occupation, looking under the surface, so as to fully examine the doing and being of humans in context.

References

Bacon, I., McKay, E.A., & Reynolds, F. (2020). The lived experience of co-dependency: An interpretative phenomenological analysis. *International Journal of Mental Health and Addiction*, 18, 754–771. https://doi.org/10.1007/s11469-018-9983-8.

Busfield, J. (1996). *Men, women and madness: Understanding gender and mental disorder.* London: Macmillan Press.

Canadian Association of Occupational Therapy (CAOT) (1997). *Enabling occupation: An occupational therapy perspective.* Ottawa: Canadian Association of Occupational Therapy.

Cooper, H. (2005). Radical exclusion: Nazi euthanasia, 1939–1945. In T. Dorrance & A. Oetzel (Eds.), *Ex Post Facto* (pp. 8–39). San Francisco: San Francisco State University.

Duncan, E., Munro, K., & Nicol, M. (2003). Research priorities in forensic occupational therapy. *British Journal of Occupational Therapy*, 66(2), 55–64.

Frank, G. (1996). Life histories in occupational therapy clinical practice. *American Journal of Occupational Therapy*, 50(4), 251–264.

Hammell, K.W. (2009). Self-care, productivity, and leisure, or dimensions of occupational experience? Rethinking occupational "categories." *Canadian Journal of Occupational Therapy*, 76(2), 107–114. https://doi.org/10.1177/000841740907600208.

Jackson, M. (1993). From work to therapy: The changing politics of occupation in the twentieth century. *British Journal of Occupational Therapy*, 56(10), 360–364.

Kemmis, S. (2009). Understanding professional practice: A synoptic framework. In B. Green (Ed.), *Understanding and Researching Professional Practice* (pp. 19–38). Rotterdam: Sense Publishers.

Kielhofner, G. (1983). *Health through occupation: Theory and practice in occupational therapy*. Philadelphia, PA: F.A. Davis.

Kielhofner, G. (1985). *A model of human occupation: Theory and application*. Baltimore, MD: Williams & Wilkins.

Kiepek, N., & Magalhães, L. (2011). Addictions and impulse-control disorders as occupation: A selected literature review and synthesis addictions and impulse-control disorders as occupation. *Journal of Occupational Science, 18*, 254–276.

Kronenberg, F., Algado, S.S., & Pollard. N. (Eds.) (2001). *Occupational therapy without borders: Learning from the spirit of survivors*. Edinburgh: Elsevier, Churchill Livingstone.

McKay, E.A. (2008). What have we been 'doing'? A historical review of occupational therapy. In E.A. McKay, C. Craik, K.H. Lim, & G. Richards (Eds.), *Advancing occupational therapy in mental health practice* (pp. 3–16). Oxford: Blackwell Publishing.

Meyer, A. (1997). The philosophy of occupational therapy. *American Journal of Occupational Therapy, 31*, 639–642 (original article 1922).

Milligan, S. (2018). Me. Retrieved from www.poemhunter.com/poem/me/.

Nicholls, L., & Elliot, M.L. (2018). In the shadow of occupation: Racism, shame and grief. *Journal of Occupational Science, 26*(3), 354–365.

Paterson, C.F. (1997). Rationales for the use of occupation in 19th century asylums. *British Journal of Occupational Therapy, 60*(4), 179–183.

Polkinghorne, D.E. (1995). Narrative configuration in qualitative analysis. *Qualitative Studies in Education, 8*(1), 5–23.

Reed, K., & Sanderson, S.R. (1980). *Concepts of occupational therapy*. Baltimore, MD: Williams & Wilkins.

Reitz, S.M. (1992). A historical review of occupational therapy's role in preventive health and wellness. *American Journal of Occupational Therapy, 46*(1), 50–55.

Townsend, E.A., & Polatajko, H.J. (2007). *Enabling occupation II: Advancing an occupational therapy vision for health, well-being, & justice through occupation*. Ottawa: CAOT Publications ACE.

Townsend, E., & Wilcock, A. (2004). Occupational justice and client-centred practice: A dialogue in progress. *Canadian Journal of Occupational Therapy, 71*(2), 75–87.

Twinley, R. (2017). The dark side of occupation. In K. Jacobs & N. MacRae (Eds.), *Occupational therapy essentials for clinical competence* (3rd ed., pp. 29–36). Thorofare, NJ: Slack.

Twinley, R., & Addidle, G. (2012). Considering violence: The dark side of occupation. *British Journal of Occupational Therapy, 75*(4), 202–204. doi:10.4276/0308022 12X13336366278257.

Whiteford, G. (2000). Occupational deprivation: Global challenge in the new millennium. *British Journal of Occupational Therapy, 63*(5), 200–204.

Whiteford, G. (2003). When people cannot participate: Occupational deprivation. In C. Christiansen & E. Townsend (Eds.), *An introduction to occupation: The art and science of living* (pp. 221–242). New Jersey: Prentice Hall.

Wilcock, A.A. (1993). A theory of the human need for occupation. *Journal of Occupational Science, 1*(1), 17–24. doi:10.1080/14427591.1993.9686375

Wilcock, A.A. (1998). *An occupational perspective of health*. Thorofare, NJ: Slack Incorporated.

Wilcock, A.A. (2001). Occupational science: The key to broadening horizons. *British Journal of Occupational Therapy*, 64(8), 412–417.

Wilcock. A.A., & Hocking, C. (2015). *An occupational perspective of health* (3rd ed.). Thorofare, NJ: Slack.

Wilcock, A.A., & Townsend, E.A. (2014). Occupational justice. In B.A. Boyt Schell, G. Gillen, M.E. Scaffa, & E.S. Cohn (Eds.), *Willard and Spackman's Occupational Therapy* (12th ed., pp. 541–552). Baltimore, MD: Lippincott Williams and Wilkins.

Yerxa, E.J., Clark, F., Frank, G., Jackson, J., Parnham, D., Pierce, D., Stein, C., & Zemke, R. (1990). An introduction to occupational science: A foundation for occupational therapy in the 21st century. *Occupational Therapy in Health Care, 6,* 1–17.

Zemke, R. & Clarke, F. (Eds.) (1996). *Occupational science: The evolving discipline.* Philadelphia, PA: F.A. Davis.

4 The whole of the moon

How our occupational lens helps or hinders our exploration of the dark side of occupation

Claire Hart

Introduction

As a discipline we have orientated ourselves towards the use of occupation to promote assumed positives. We assert the potential of occupation to provide purpose, structure, achievement, pleasure, social connectedness, identity, and well-being (Hasselkus, 2011; Holahan, 2014; Leufstadius, Erlandsson, Björkman, & Eklund, 2011; Whalley Hammell, 2015, Wildschut & Meyer, 2016). In a discourse all about positive occupation and positive outcomes there may be little space to hear alternative experiences of occupation, or see the negative influence of occupational injustice on true occupational choice.

This call to explore the dark side of occupation is an opportunity to explore how new professional insights chime with our existing body of knowledge. However valuable this may be, there are always barriers to attending to and representing new concepts (Samuelsson & Wressle, 2015). Adopting new ideas requires us to have a focused understanding of the issues and context, the values and beliefs of all involved, and the communication channels used to promote change (Burke & Gitlin, 2012). In addressing the dark side of occupation, we face new and unfamiliar ideas and a challenge to accepted norms on occupation. As with any fledgling concept, the dark side of occupation is still being debated and refined, and there are different voices and interpretations to be heard. The ideas we explore may contest some fundamental professional beliefs and challenge us on the scope of our practice. We must also face our natural reluctance to explore the unknown, turning our attention to unfamiliar, and sometimes uncomfortable, aspects of occupational life.

Moustakas (1990) describes discovering new ideas and concepts as somewhat like finding an empty seat in a dark theatre. It requires us to tolerate darkness and unfamiliarity, using whatever information we can to feel our way and find where we need to be. This chapter acknowledges the discomfort of the unfamiliar, dark spaces associated with the unknown, and the quality of the information we have to guide us.

Seeing the whole of the moon

Before we act on any concept we must first *see* it. Twinley describes the dark side of occupation as like the dark side of the moon, something unseen that needs to be explored in order to be understood (Twinley, 2013, 2017). We cannot begin to observe the totality of occupation unless we give it our full, critical attention, and at present our professional attentions are drawn in many different directions.

Intentionality is the power of the mind to attend to and represent ideas (Guerin, 2013; Jacob, 2019), and it is key to the development of understanding and knowledge (Hopp, 2011). The ability to attend fully to things and direct "intentionality" is increasingly acknowledged as essential to understanding the lived experience of occupation (Park Lala & Kinsella, 2011; Pickens & Pizur-Barnekow, 2009; Ramugondo & Kronenberg, 2013). There is growing recognition that we need to understand intentionality in relation to the meaning and motivation behind people's occupational choices (Pickens & Pizur-Barnekow, 2009; Ramugondo & Kronenberg, 2013), and I would argue this is particularly important in understanding their engagement with the dark side of occupation.

However, intentionality also helps us to understand concepts and issues faced in our own professional practice (Carlson, Portman, & Bartlett, 2011; Putnam, Smith, & Cassady, 2009). Nevertheless, just "looking" may not be enough. Intentionality has the potential to be inquisitive and exploratory or fixed and incurious (Greene & Brown, 2009; Turner, 2017). We can easily turn our attention only to those things we already know and understand, or those with which we are comfortably familiar. We need to give conscious and deliberate consideration to areas of practice that may be ill-understood to improve our understanding of the nature of the occupation and its role in the lives of others. The real value in intentionality lies in our ability to look around and be critical (Carlson, Portman, & Bartlett, 2011; Putnam, Smith, & Cassady, 2009).

To fully *see* occupation we must incorporate the dark side, and see the "whole of the moon". However, we cannot do that unless we direct our intentionality towards it. *Seeing* means being clear about the concepts being explored, being open about our professional positionality and being willing to explore new ideas about people's occupational lives. At present we may not be directing our intentionality towards the dark side of occupation for a number of reasons: the newness of the concept; the desire to look to the positive; our fear of the unknown; and a lack of direction from within existing theory. All of these features are part of the wider "occupational lens" we use to explore practice issues, they create the context and enable or prevent us from addressing issues.

Seeing and agreeing the concept

Interest in the concept of the dark side of occupation appears to be growing, with an increase in exploration and dialogue by practitioners, academics, and researchers. The concept has been met with enthusiasm, lively debate, and some controversy; all of which suggests a healthy discourse, necessary during the early stages of a developing concept.

One notable issue in exploring the premise of the dark side of occupation, lies in the language used to capture the concept and discuss it within the discipline. There is often a lot of debate about the suitability of terms used and the parameters of new definitions, and as the dark side of occupation is a concept in its relative infancy, discussions are evolving in similar but different ways in different parts of the world. For example, academic and practice staff from Canada are presenting similar themes under the title "non-sanctioned occupations" (Illman et al., 2013; Kiepek, Beagan, Laliberte Rudman, & Phelan, 2019). This is described as activities framed as "unhealthy", "deviant", and illegal, with recognition that external perspectives shape societal views of the occupations of others (Kiepek et al., 2019). Significant similarities exist between this and perspectives on the dark side of occupation introduced earlier by Twinley and Addidle (2012) and Twinley (2013, 2017). Each perspective draws attention to occupational therapy's explicit focus on the positive nature of occupation, both identify the potential of a broader understanding of occupation to illuminate the client's unique frame of reference, and both challenge the profession on its value judgements and moral positioning (Kiepek et al., 2019; Twinley, 2017).

Both terms have received significant attention, suggesting they have value in our ongoing exploration of occupation, but both have also received a degree of criticism. Some people fear that the "dark side of occupation" suggests that occupations may be inherently "dark" or "light", though this is clarified in Chapters 1 and 2, and some see the term "non-sanctioned occupation" as somewhat all-or-nothing, or focused more on the perspective of the external observer. However, my personal perspective is that terminology reflects the different origins of the term, and different language preferences in North America and the UK have shaped these ideas more than conceptual difference. Neither term is perfect, but they are part of a fledgling attempt to understand raw concepts that have previously been unnamed.

This discourse should not be seen as a negative, as discussions on ideas and terminology are a valuable part of our profession's reflective process. It is what Bourdieu termed "epistemic reflexivity" (Bourdieu & Wacquant, 1992; Kinsella & Whiteford, 2009), where we explore in order to gain a greater understanding of the assumptions and ideas that underpin our theory and practice. Understanding our history, philosophy, and stance on key issues is part of ensuring our actions are consistent with our core values (Kinsella & Whiteford, 2009; Yerxa, 1992), but also a means of acknowledging the uniqueness (Townsend & Polatajko, 2013) and maturity of our discipline (Kinsella & Whiteford, 2009).

Having a discourse and challenging ideas is not necessarily about reaching a universal understanding, but is an opportunity to engage with a reflective process and explore our contemporary position (Kinsella & Whiteford, 2009; Vasilachis de Gialdino, 2009). After all, ambiguity and lack of consensus are a natural part of the layered complexity of occupation (Müllersdorf & Ivarsson, 2010). I would suggest that there is space in the development of these ideas for more than one strand of thinking, and that attempting to close routes of exploration at this stage could limit concept development.

Keeping to the positives

The second major challenge to exploring the dark side of occupation lies in our ongoing investment in the positive nature of occupation. The value of occupation forms a fundamental part of the ethos and philosophy of occupational therapy and occupational science, and many of the benefits of occupation are well established and incontrovertible (Alnervik & Linddahl, 2011). We have highlighted the capacity of occupation to influence well-being (Whalley Hammell & Iwama, 2012), improve the human condition (Wilcock, 2006), and directly affect health (Durocher, Gibson, & Rappolt, 2013).

Through time, our focus on the centrality of occupation has waxed and waned (Wong & Fisher, 2015). However, by emphasising its gains and potential, we have encouraged others to see the inherent value of occupation-based interventions as "one of the great ideas of 20th Century medicine" (Reilly, 1961, p. 1). This, in part, reflects a fervent belief in occupation, but perhaps also our ongoing battle to assert our value as a profession. Occupation has always been our Unique Selling Point, and we have sold occupation to our peers, our clients, and ourselves on the basis of its many positives.

I should be clear that I do not disagree with this stance, but I recognise it as the polished view for public consumption. Behind this "marketing" of occupation, and occupational therapy, there is a need to acknowledge that occupations, like the people who perform them, are complex and messy.

Our propensity to focus on the positives of occupation may not seem problematic, but it has meant that our intentionality is directed towards a particular occupational focus. We have looked at occupations where they are health-promoting or socially accepted, without acknowledging the true range of occupations chosen by the individual or made available to them (Durocher, Gibson & Rappolt, 2013; Townsend, 2015; van Bruggen, 2014).

There are increasing calls for the profession to let go of some of the "culturally specific, class-bound, and ableist" (Whalley Hammell, 2009, p. 107) views of occupation and focus instead on recognition of occupations on the basis of their value to the individual (Jonsson, 2008). By focusing more on the lived experience of occupation (Whalley Hammell, 2015), the nature of the occupation per se (Hocking, 2009), the motivation toward the occupation (Reed, Hocking, & Smythe, 2010) or the contextual influences on the occupation (Dickie, Cutchin, & Humphry, 2006), we gain far greater insight into its meaning. This does not mean turning our intentionality away from the potential of occupation, but looking more deeply and wholly in order to fully "see" the occupational life of the client.

Fear of the unknown and uncomfortable

Many of us became therapists because we wanted to improve the lives of others, and seeing people move in ways that do not support their health or well-being can be extremely disheartening (Serani, 2011; Werbart et al., 2014). Just as Cunningham and Pace highlight in Chapter 19, building rapport, trust, and understanding can be challenging; our humanity may help us to forge empathy, but it may also bring our own values and morality into the therapeutic relationship (Law et al., 1996; Sumsion & Smyth, 2000). It takes courage to trust the client's own process and follow their lead when we don't fully understand it, fear it, or even disapprove of it (Rogers, 1951). Effective use of self involves being aware of our own interpersonal reactions to and expectations of clients, including those who may challenge these through what we might perceive as negative behaviour (Taylor, 2020).

Rogers (1951, 1980) identified the essential role of acceptance and understanding within the many uncomfortable stages of the therapeutic process, without which the individual has no safe place to share and no sense that their lived experience can be understood. Our propensity to focus on the positive can prevent us from directing our attention towards other aspects, and if our agenda with our clients is all about "the right kind of occupation" we may unconsciously prevent people from exposing aspects of their occupational lives which they fear we may disapprove of.

The more we disattend to behaviours we dislike, fear, or do not understand, the more this can cause the client to dissociate from them, and the more hidden and forbidden they become (Henderson, 2018). As Jung said, "everyone carries a shadow, and the less it is embodied in the individual's conscious life, the blacker and denser it is" (Jung, 1938, p. 131).

Our occupational lens

Practice has long been dominated by a few key models, mostly encapsulating North American perspectives on occupation. The arrival of the Model of Human Occupation (MOHO) (Kielhofner, 1980) provided an opportunity to better understand how occupation is motivated, patterned, and performed (Kielhofner, 2008). A number of subsequent models have reflected both the nature of human occupations and occupational therapy practice (Occupational Performance Model (Australia), Chapparo & Ranka, 1997). They have increased the focus on context (Ecology of Human Performance, Dunn, Brown, & McGuigan, 1994), environment (Person-Environment-Occupation Model, Law et al., 1996), or client perspective (Canadian Model of Occupational Performance, CAOT 1997). More latterly, the Vona du Toit Model of Creative Ability (VdTMoCA) (De Witt, 2014) from South Africa, and the Kawa Model (Iwama, 2006) from Japan, attempted to introduce alternative voices from other communities of therapists (Ashby & Chandler, 2010).

Models of practice provide a theoretical backdrop which attempts to capture the complex and multifaceted nature of occupation, and direct practitioners to the value of occupation to their clients (Erlandsson, Eklund, & Persson, 2009; Maclean, Carin-Levy, Hunter, Malcolmson, & Locke, 2012). Models can help us to locate our practice in a guiding framework, from which we must look and reason in order to apply the model to the individual client before us (Youngstrom, 2012).

There does not appear to be an explicit place within existing models of practice which directs the user to focus on the dark side of occupation. However, it is appropriate to acknowledge that as a fledgling concept, the dark side of occupation is something that the profession is only beginning to acknowledge. As a result, we would be unlikely to find this unknown, unacknowledged, messy, and complex aspect of occupation embedded in theory which significantly pre-dates it.

The potential and challenge associated with using occupational therapy models in this field is possibly a reflection of the use of models per se. The value of theoretical and practice models is well established (Wong & Fisher, 2015). Models have been central to establishing a theory base and creating a lexicon for practice, academia, and research (Boniface & Seymour, 2012; Duncan, 2020). The occupation-focused nature of our models provides an essential vehicle for articulating our core professional contribution (Joosten, 2015; Turpin & Iwama, 2011).

However, the application of models is not without challenge (Wong & Fisher, 2015). Despite having a wide range of models available to us, their use is sporadic and not always driven by the pursuit of practice outcomes (Ashby & Chandler, 2010; Owen, Adams, & Franszen, 2014). Therapists choose their model through an interplay between their own characteristics and the demands of their workplace (Owen, Adams, & Franszen, 2014). Educational background, experience, exposure in the clinical field, and the ethos of their workplace, practical constraints, and client need all shape model choice (Owen, Adams, & Franszen, 2014; Wong & Fisher, 2015). Models are not always applied consistently and systematically due to limited understanding of underpinning theory, creating a significant gap remaining between theory and practice (Ikuigu & Smallfield, 2011; Nash & Mitchell, 2017).

In addition, there are limited voices shaping the field of models, with MOHO and CMOP-Engagement remaining dominant in practice and education, despite new models emerging (Ashby & Chandler, 2010). This maintains the reliance on these models and the power of key, Western, voices (Ashby & Chandler, 2010; Turpin & Iwama, 2011).

Third, there are debates about the capacity for models to wholly represent occupational lives (Haglund & Kjelberg, 1999; Hocking, 1994). The more complex the circumstances the harder it is to develop a model that reflects the multi-layered issues faced (Jahan & Ellibidy, 2017). Occupation is accepted as inherently complex (Müllersdorf & Ivarsson, 2010; Pentland, Kantartzis, Giatsi Clausen, & Witemyre, 2018), and there have been many attempts to capture, define, and categorise occupation in order to reduce ambiguity and make concepts more manageable (Hocking & Wright-St. Clair, 2011; Whalley Hammell, 2015). However, increasingly we are encouraged to tolerate the complexity and embrace models which reflect broader patterns of occupational awareness and lived experience (Hocking, 2009; Whalley Hammell, 2015; Wong & Fisher, 2015).

There is a parallel here with the challenge of understanding the dark side of occupation. We have an uncomfortable, unknown, and complex phenomenon, and may be seeking to apply simple conceptual frameworks to understand it. As Jahan and Ellibidy (2017) stated, models will often struggle to apply to complex lives or needs.

Meeting the complex, unknown, or challenging in practice often encourages us to reach for something simple or prescriptive to help us to understand it (Owen, 2014). This is particularly the case if we are novices to the profession, or to a particular field of practice (Standing, 2010).

Simple practice issues are like baking a cake: follow the recipe and most people can anticipate a degree of success. You cannot, however, use a basic recipe to make a space rocket; you need more technical information, training, and specialist skills, so your model would need greater depth and you would need more significant training. For complex issues, even technical information and training may be insufficient. Complex practice issues are more like raising a child. You need skills, knowledge, and wisdom, and may have many conflicting sources of guidance – and even then, there are no guarantees of success.

We cannot take a simple recipe to the complex, messy, ill-understood aspects of the dark side of occupation. In complex lives we may need to employ "wise practice" or "knowing practice" (Higgs, 2016), where practitioners use a mixture of types of evidence, including tacit knowledge and practical wisdom (Blair & Robertson, 2005). It is acknowledged that with experience many practitioners "work beyond" their chosen models to enable them to work with complexity (Owen, Adams, & Franszen, 2014;

Ikuigu & Smallfield, 2011). In complex circumstances we may need to keep an open mind (Owen, Adams & Franszen, 2014), focus more on "possibilities-based practice" (Kronenberg, Pollard, & Sakellariou, 2011) and "wise practice" (Higgs, 2016), and be ready to use existing and invaluable models as a firm footing from which to explore (Vasilachis de Gialdino, 2009).

Whilst no model makes a specific attempt to direct practitioners to consider the dark side of occupation, it is eminently possible to use existing models to capture client experiences of a wide range of occupations. For example, if a model can help us to explore the dynamic between facets that influence occupational performance, it can do so for any occupation. The challenge in exploring the dark side may be its unfamiliarity or complexity. It isn't the model that may be ill-equipped, but our ability to approach its use in more challenging fields (Ikuigu & Smallfield, 2011; Owen, Adams, & Franszen, 2014). The potential is there in any model to identify the meaning, function, and experience of the dark side of occupation, but only if the therapist is looking in that direction. Cole and Tufano (2008) assert that our approach to models requires a particular "reasoning", an open and enquiring exploration of the models to choose on the basis of suitability and "best fit". The job of choosing lies with the therapist, no model can make you look where you need to, that is a matter of insight and intentionality.

Conclusions: lens and mirror

Our occupational theory presents us with opportunities to look outward and understand occupational lives with greater depth, and inwardly to hold a mirror to our profession. Intentionality reminds us to look, look widely, and look with openness and curiosity. We must direct our intentionality at a breadth of occupations, a breadth of people and, critically, back towards ourselves.

It is a long-held belief that understanding others starts first with understanding oneself (Andonian, 2017; Hagedorn, 1995; Mosey, 1986). We must first reflect on how our personal and professional perspectives will shape our view of the dark side of occupation. In this context we require not only self-awareness, but also "profession-awareness" showing our understanding of how our epistemological position shapes our world view (Kinsella & Whiteford, 2009; Townsend & Polatajko, 2013).

We cannot be truly holistic, client-centred, and occupation-focused without acknowledging a broad range of occupations as experienced by a broad range of individuals (Twinley, 2017). Unchallenged, our theory base could impose perspectives on "ideal" ways of living (Al Busaidy & Borthwick, 2012; Kantartzis & Molineux, 2011), or focus only on the occupations that support our idea of positivity, productivity, and health (Pierce, 2012). This has negative political, practical, and theoretical implications (Castro, Dahlin-Ivanoff, & Mårtensson, 2014), and reduces our potential to be inclusive and socially relevant (Pierce, 2012; Twinley & Addidle, 2012).

The discourse on the dark side of occupation, and other similar movements in the development of the profession, can create a theoretical bridge by using an additional lens (Nilsson & Townsend, 2010). Maybe the question is not what the models tell us about the dark side of occupation, but what the dark side of occupation can do to inform and stretch the application of our existing theory base? Arguably, no model can capture every facet of every occupational life, or direct the therapist towards every conceivable field of interest – models are merely shaping our field of vision, and it is up to us to decide where to look. A model might provide us with a lens, but again we have to be aware enough to look in multiple directions; and be ready to "see".

References

Al Busaidy, N.S.M., & Borthwick, A. (2012). Occupational therapy in Oman: The impact of cultural dissonance. *Occupational Therapy International*, *19*, pp. 154–164.

Alnervik, A., & Linddahl, I. (2011). Value of occupational therapy – about evidence-based occupational therapy. *Nacka: Förbundet Sveriges Arbetsterapeuter*. Retrieved from: http://urn.kb.se/resolve?urn=urn:nbn:se:hj:diva-15557.

Andonian, L. (2017). Emotional intelligence: An opportunity for occupational therapy. *Occupational Therapy in Mental Health*, *33*(4), pp. 299–307.

Ashby, S., & Chandler, B. (2010). An exploratory study of the occupation-focused models included in occupational therapy professional education programmes. *British Journal of Occupational Therapy*, *73*(12), pp. 616–624.

Blair, S.E.E., & Robertson, L.J. (2005). Hard complexities – soft complexities: An exploration of philosophical positions related to evidence in occupational therapy. *British Journal of Occupational Therapy*, *68*(6), pp. 269–276.

Boniface, G., & Seymour, A. (Eds.) (2012). *Using occupational therapy theory in practice*. Oxford: Wiley-Blackwell.

Bourdieu, P., & Waquant, L.D.J. (1992). *An Invitation to Reflexive Sociology*. Chicago: University of Chicago Press.

Burke, J.P., & Gitlin, L.N. (2012). The issue is: How do we change practice when we have the evidence? *American Journal of Occupational Therapy*, *66*, pp. 85–88.

Carlson, L.A., Portman, T.A.A., & Bartlett, J.R. (2011). Self-management of career development: Intentionality for counselor educators in training. *Journal of Humanistic Counselling*, *45*(2), pp. 126–137.

Castro, D., Dahlin-Ivanoff, S., & Mårtensson, L. (2014). Occupational therapy and culture: A literature review. *Scandinavian Journal of Occupational Therapy*, *21*(6), pp. 401–414.

Chapparo, C., & Ranka, J. (1997). Occupational Performance Model (Australia): Monograph 1. OP Network, The University of Sydney.

Cole, M., & Tufano, R. (2008). *Applied theories in occupational therapy: A practical approach*. Thorofare, NJ: Slack.

De Witt, P. (2014). Creative ability: A model for individual and group occupational therapy for clients with psychosocial dysfunction. In R. Crouch & V. Alers (Eds.), *Occupational therapy in psychiatry and mental health* (5th ed., pp. 3–32). London and Philadelphia: Whurr Publishers.

Dickie, V., Cutchin, M., & Humphry, R. (2006). Occupation as transactional experience: A critique of individualism in occupational science. *Journal of Occupational Science, 13*(1), pp. 83–93.

Duncan, E.A.S. (Ed.) (2020). *Foundations for practice in occupational therapy* (6th ed.). London: Elsevier.

Dunn, W., Brown, C., & McGuigan, A. (1994). The ecology of human performance: A framework for considering the effect of context. *American Journal of Occupational Therapy, 48*(7), pp. 595–607.

Durocher, E., Gibson, B.E., & Rappolt, S. (2013). Occupational justice: A conceptual review. *Journal of Occupational Science, 21*(4), pp. 418–430.

Erlandsson, L.-K., Eklund, M., & Persson, D. (2009). Occupational value and relationships to meaning and health: Elaborations of the ValMO-model. *Scandinavian Journal of Occupational Therapy, 18*(1), pp. 72–80.

Greene, J., & Brown, S. (2009). The Wisdom Development Scale: Further validity investigations. *International Journal of Aging Human Development, 68*, pp. 289–320.

Guerin, M. (2013). Intentionality. Retrieved from https://politicalanthro.wordpress.com/intentionality/.

Hagedorn, R. (1995). The Casson Memorial Lecture 1995: An emergent profession – a personal perspective. *British Journal of Occupational Therapy, 58*(8), pp. 324–331.

Haglund, L., & Kjelberg, A. (1999). A critical analysis of the Model of Human Occupation. *Canadian Journal of Occupational Therapy, 66*(2), pp. 102–108.

Hasselkus, B.R. (2011). *The meaning of everyday occupation*. Thorofare, NJ: Slack.

Henderson, J.L. (2018). *Shadow and self: Selected papers in analytical psychology*. Asheville, NC: Chiron Publications.

Higgs, J. (2016). Practice wisdom and wise practice. In J. Higgs & F. Trede (Eds.), *Professional practice discourse marginalia. Practice, education, work and society* (pp. 65–72). Rotterdam: Sense Publishers.

Hocking, C. (1994). Objects in the environment: A critique of the Model of Human Occupation dimensions. *Scandinavian Journal of Occupational Therapy, 1*(2), pp. 77–84. doi:10.3109/11038129409106666.

Hocking, C. (2009). The challenge of occupation: Describing the things people do. *Journal of Occupational Science, 16*(3), pp. 140–150. doi:10.1080/14427591.2009.9686655.

Hocking, C., & Wright-St. Clair, V. (2011). Occupational science: Adding value to occupational therapy. *New Zealand Journal of Occupational Therapy, 58*(1), pp. 29–35.

Holahan, L.F. (2014). Quality-in-doing: Competence and occupation. *Journal of Occupational Science, 21*(4), pp. 473–487.

Hopp, W. (2011). *Perception and knowledge: A phenomenological account*. Cambridge: Cambridge University Press.

Illman, S.C., Spence, S., O'Campo, P., & Kirsh, B. (2013). Exploring the occupations of homeless adults living with mental illnesses in Toronto. *Canadian Journal of Occupational Therapy, 80*(4), pp. 215–223.

Ikiugu, M.N., & Smallfield, S. (2011). Ikiugu's eclectic method of combining theoretical conceptual practice models in occupational therapy. *Australian Occupational Therapy Journal, 58*(6), pp. 437–446.

Iwama, M. (2006). *The Kawa Model: Culturally relevant occupational therapy*. Philadelphia: Churchill Livingstone.

Jacob, P. (2019). Intentionality. In E.N. Zalta (Ed.), *The Stanford encyclopedia of philosophy* (Winter 2019 ed.). Retrieved from: https://plato.stanford.edu/archives/win2019/entries/intentionality/.

Jahan, A., & Ellibidy, A. (2017). A review of conceptual models for rehabilitation research and practice. *Journal of Rehabilitation Sciences, 2*, pp. 46–53.

Jonsson, H. (2008). A new direction in the conceptualization and categorization of occupation. *Journal of Occupational Science, 15*(38), pp. 3–8.

Joosten, A.V. (2015). Contemporary occupational therapy: Our occupational therapy models are essential to occupation centred practice. *Australian Occupational Therapy Journal, 62*(3), pp. 219–222.

Jung, C.G. (1938). *Psychology and religion.* New Haven, CT: Yale University Press.

Kantartzis, S., & Molineux, M. (2011). The influence of Western society's construction of a healthy daily life on the conceptualisation of occupation. *Journal of Occupational Science, 18*(1), pp. 62–80.

Kielhofner, G. (2008). *Model of human occupation: Theory and application* (4th ed.). Baltimore: Lippincott, Williams & Wilkins.

Kiepek, N., Beagan, B., Laliberte Rudman, D., & Phelan, S. (2019). Silences around occupations framed as unhealthy, illegal, and deviant. *Journal of Occupational Science, 26*(3), 341–353. doi:10.1080/14427591.2018.1499123.

Kinsella, E.A., & Whiteford, G. (2009). Knowledge generation and utilization: Toward epistemic reflexivity. *Australian Occupational Therapy Journal, 56*(4), pp. 249–258.

Kronenberg, F., Pollard, N., & Sakellariou, D. (Eds.) (2011). *Occupational therapies without borders: Vol. 2 Towards an ecology of occupation-based practice.* Edinburgh: Churchill Livingstone.

Law, M., Cooper, B., Strong, J., Stewart, D., Rigby, P., & Letts, L. (1996). The person-environment-occupation model: A transactive approach to occupational performance. *Canadian Journal of Occupational Therapy, 63*(1), pp. 9–23.

Leufstadius, C., Erlandsson, L.-K., Björkman T., & Eklund, M. (2011). Meaningfulness in daily occupations among individuals with persistent mental illness. *Journal of Occupational Science, 15*(1), pp. 27–35.

Maclean, F., Carin-Levy, G., Hunter, H., Malcolmson, L., & Locke, E. (2012). The usefulness of the Person-Environment-Occupation Model (PEO Model) in an acute physical health care setting. *British Journal of Occupational Therapy, 75*(12), pp. 1–8.

Mosey, A.C. (1986). *The psychosocial components of occupational therapy.* New York: Raven Press.

Moustakas, C. (1990). *Heuristic research: Design, methodology and applications.* Newbury Park, CA: Sage.

Müllersdorf, M., & Ivarsson, A.B. (2010). Use of creative activities in occupational therapy practice in Sweden. *Occupational Therapy International, 19*(3), pp. 127–134.

Nash, B.H., & Mitchell, A.W. (2017). Longitudinal study of changes in occupational therapy students' perspectives on frames of reference. *American Journal of Occupational Therapy, 71*(5), 7105230010. https://doi.org/10.5014/ajot.2017.024455.

Nilsson, I., & Townsend, E. (2010). Occupational justice – bridging theory and practice. *Scandinavian Journal of Occupational Therapy, 17*(1), pp. 57–63.

Owen, A. (2014). Model use in occupational therapy practice with a focus on the Kawa model. Retrieved from https://core.ac.uk/download/pdf/39674030.pdf?repositoryId=979.

Owen, A., Adams, F., & Franszen, D. (2014). Factors influencing model use in occupational therapy. *South African Journal of Occupational Therapy, 44*(1), pp. 41–47.

Park Lala, A., & Kinsella, E.A. (2011). Phenomenology and the study of human occupation. *Journal of Occupational Science*, 18(3), pp. 195–209.

Pentland, D., Kantartzis, S., Giatsi Clausen, M., & Witemyre, K. (2018). *Occupational therapy and complexity: Defining and describing practice*. London: Royal College of Occupational Therapists.

Pickens, N.D., & Pizur-Barnekow, K. (2009). Co-occupation: Extending the dialogue. *Journal of Occupational Science*, 16(3), pp. 151–156. doi:10.1080/14427591.2 009.9686656.

Pierce, D. (2012). Promise. *Journal of Occupational Science*, 19(4), pp. 298–311.

Putnam, M., Smith, L.L., & Cassady, J.C. (2009). Promoting change through professional development: The place of teacher intentionality in reading instruction. *Literacy Research and Instruction*, 48(3), pp. 207–220.

Ramugondo, E.L., & Kronenberg, F. (2013). Explaining collective occupations from a human relations perspective: Bridging the individual-collective dichotomy. *Journal of Occupational Science*, 22(1), pp. 3–16.

Reed, K., Hocking, C.S., & Smythe, L.A. (2010). The interconnected meanings of occupation: The call, being-with, possibilities. *Journal of Occupational Science*, 17(3), pp. 140–149.

Reilly, M. (1961). The 1961 Eleanor Clarke Slagle Lecture. Occupational therapy can be one of the great ideas of 20th century medicine. *American Journal of Occupational Therapy*, 16(1), pp. 87–105.

Rogers, C.R. (1951). *Client-centered therapy: Its current practice, implications and theory*. Boston: Houghton Mifflin.

Rogers, C.R. (1980). *A way of being*. New York: Houghton Mifflin.

Samuelsson, K., & Wressle, E. (2015). Turning evidence into practice: Barriers to research use among occupational therapists. *British Journal of Occupational Therapy*, 78(3), pp. 175–181.

Serani, D. (2011). *Living with depression: Why biology and biography matter along the path to hope and healing*. Lanham, MD: Rowman & Littlefield Publishers.

Standing, M. (2010). *Clinical judgement and decision-making in nursing and interprofessional healthcare*. Maidenhead: McGraw Hill.

Sumsion, T., & Smyth, G. (2000). Barriers to client-centredness and their resolution. *Canadian Journal of Occupational Therapy*, 67(1), pp. 15–21.

Taylor, R.R. (2020). *The intentional relationship: Occupational therapy and use of self*. Philadelphia: F.A. Davis Company.

Townsend, E.A. (2015). The 2014 Ruth Zemke Lectureship in Occupational Science. Critical occupational literacy: Thinking about occupational justice, ecological sustainability, and aging in everyday life. *Journal of Occupational Science*, 22(4), pp. 389–402. doi:10.1080/14427591.2015.1071691.

Townsend, E.A., & Polatajko, H.J. (2013). *Enabling occupation II: Advancing an occupational therapy vision for health, well-being, and justice through occupation* (2nd ed.) Ottawa: CAOT Publications ACE.

Turner, C.K. (2017). A principal of intentionality. *Frontiers in Psychology*, 8, p. 137.

Turpin, M., & Iwama, M. (2011). *Using occupational therapy models in practice: A field guide*. Edinburgh: Elsevier.

Twinley, R. (2013). The dark side of occupation: A concept for consideration. *Australian Occupational Therapy Journal*, 60(4), pp. 301–303. doi:10.1111/1440-1630. 12026.

Twinley, R. (2017). The dark side of occupation. In K. Jacobs & N. MacRae (Eds.), *Occupational therapy essentials for clinical competence* (3rd ed., pp. 29–36). Thorofare, NJ: Slack.

Twinley, R., and Addidle, G. (2012). Considering violence: The dark side of occupation. *British Journal of Occupational Therapy*, 75(4), pp. 202–204. doi:10.4276/03 0802212X13336366278257.

van Bruggen, H. (2014). Turning challenges into opportunities: How occupational therapy is contributing to social, health and educational reform. *World Federation of Occupational Therapists Bulletin*, 70(1), pp. 41–46.

Vasilachis de Gialdino, I. (2009). Ontological and epistemological foundations of qualitative research. *Forum Qualitative Sozialforschung/Forum: Qualitative Social Research*, 10(2), Art. 30. http://dx.doi.org/10.17169/fqs-10.2.1299.

Werbart, A., von Below, C., Brun, J., & Gunnarsdottir, H. (2014). "Spinning one's wheels": Nonimproved patients view their psychotherapy. *Psychotherapy Research*, 25(5), pp. 1–19.

Whalley Hammell, K. (2009). Self-care, productivity, and leisure, or dimensions of occupational experience? Rethinking occupational "categories". *Canadian Journal of Occupational Therapy*, 76(2), pp. 107–14.

Whalley Hammell, K. (2015). Quality of life, participation and occupational rights: A capabilities perspective. *Australian Occupational Therapy Journal*, 62(2), pp. 78–85.

Whalley Hammell, K., & Iwama, M.K. (2012). Well-being and occupational rights: An imperative for critical occupational therapy. *Scandinavian Journal of Occupational Therapy*, 19(5), pp. 385–394.

Wilcock, A.A. (2006). *An Occupational Perspective of Health* (2nd ed.). Thorofare, NJ: Slack.

Wildschut, A., & Meyer, T. (2016). The shifting boundaries of artisanal work and occupations. Labour Market Intelligence Partnership. Retrieved from www.lmip.org. za/sites/default/files/documentfiles/504.%20The%20Shifting%20Boundaries%20 of%20Artisanal%20Work%20And%20Occupations_0.pdf.

Wong, S.R., & Fisher, G. (2015). Comparing and using occupation-focused models. *Occupational Therapy in Health Care*, 29(3), pp. 297–315.

Yerxa, E.J. (1992). Some implications of occupational therapy's history for its epistemology, values, and relation to medicine. *American Journal of Occupational Therapy*, 46(1), pp. 79–83.

Youngstrom, M. (2012). The occupational therapy practice framework: The evolution of our professional language. *American Journal of Occupational Therapy*, 56(6), pp. 607–608.

5 Ontological and epistemological considerations in understanding occupations in extreme and/or oppressive contexts

"Doing non-violent resistance" in Palestine

Gail Whiteford and Aliya Haddad

Background

Human occupation is always situated and inherently complex. Whiteford, Jones, Rahal, and Suleman (2018), in their work on the Participatory Occupational Justice Framework, suggest that:

> All occupation takes place in a context. That is, no human action is independent of the social, cultural, political and economic contexts in which it occurs. These contextual forces, to a greater or lesser extent, shape the form and performance of the occupation as well as the meaning ascribed to it by an individual or group. Contextual influences can include the prevailing economic ideologies and related policies, cultural and faith-based systems that govern social and occupational behaviour, health and social network supports, educational systems and structures, use of social media, telecommunications and transportation and environmental protections as well as primary resource management.
>
> (p. 4)

Developing understandings of this complex rubric within which occupation takes place and the causal relationships that exist and exert a powerful influence, not only on form and performance but also on legitimacy and opportunity, obviously represents a significant challenge. Occupational science research has been oriented towards growing our understandings of occupation as a complex, situated phenomenon and, to date, the corpus of research on occupation has grown, undertaken by researchers around the globe (Molineux & Whiteford, in press). As many of these researchers have argued over time, however, the dynamism of occupation cannot be captured through experimental means. Accordingly, research approaches which seek to illuminate the ontological and epistemological perspectives – or, put more simply, the realities and ways of knowing – of people in different contexts as they engage in a myriad of occupations, have been argued as most appropriate and, indeed, most ethical (Ramugondo, 2015).

The ultimate value of occupational science, however, will be realised through its ability to generate new and useful knowledge as judged by its stakeholders. Relevancy has overwhelmingly become the concern of not just stakeholders but funders, academics, and practitioners alike when they discuss research (Durocher, Gibson & Rappolt, 2014). This represents a timely and appropriate response when, at worst, many abuses of intellectual and human rights have historically occurred in the name of research and, at best, research has been compromised in its usefulness by a lack of regard for application in real-world contexts. This means including consideration of the historic, political, and economic factors shaping access and participation for whole groups of people and the discursive traditions that influence policy development (Molineux & Whiteford, in press). In essence, it means advancing epistemic alongside occupational justice (Fricker, 2007).

As suggested above, the opportunity to enact epistemic justice as a response to protracted, historical scenarios in which people have been unable to effectively "have a voice", is part of the broader social contract of universities globally. For this reason, the authors developed a research proposal aiming at exploring the experiences and constructed meanings of people living in Palestine as they engaged in forms of everyday, non-violent resistance. Once ethics approval was gained at a university in Palestine, convenience and snowball sampling strategies were employed to recruit staff and student participants for semi-structured interviews in places of their choosing. Interviews were conducted with an existential, phenomenological intent (Liamputtong, 2013), that is, to attempt to illuminate the lived experience of non-violent resistance and its associated meanings for people in everyday life.

Following open coding and the generation of provisional themes, an ongoing dialogue between the researchers has developed in order to understand the narrative data relative to context. In order to further understandings of how we can begin to understand this construction from ontological and epistemological standpoints – that is, from the perspective of those whose everyday realities, knowledges and identities are impacted – we have developed three theoretical propositions for consideration. These propositions are informed by the narrative data generated in the study and are supported by data extracts and relate to: ontological, epistemological, and representational considerations. Due to size constraints of this chapter, we are only presenting the first two for consideration with a limited amount of interpretive commentary so as to award the narrative data primacy of representation.

> **Proposition 1:** In order to understand aspects of *being in* and respond-ing to oppressive/limiting conditions, it is important to understand the person(s)' lived reality or ontological *standpoint*. In order to do this we need to illuminate specific features of the environments and contexts in which they live.

Put yourself in our shoes: attempting ontological understandings of extreme conditions

> There is a poem in Arabic that means if I took out both your eyes and replaced them with diamonds, would you see again? It means people do not see the suffering, people are losing their homes, their lives, their families and it is not easy to accept. People need to experience – to put themselves in our shoes to really know the reality of our life.
>
> We are second class citizens, everything is much harder. Like wanting to work and there is not time because your time is taken away from you in moving around. We have lower income and that stops us doing things.

The reflections above point to what the participants in this study want the reader to know and understand. First, that they feel like second class citizens in the context of being and living in the occupied territories and the multitude of impacts on everyday life; and, second, that it is such an extreme existence in which suffering occurs on a daily basis that it has to be appreciated directly.

The biggest single barrier is the checkpoint: physical conditions and political barriers which limit access and participation

Many people – individuals and families – live in suboptimal conditions in Palestine due to the restricted choice they have in *where* they can live. For this reason, overcrowding is not uncommon in some areas.

> We were in a one room home for years, four children and our parents – with mould and water coming in. My mum hates winter and we lived with mould for years, we all had fights but had to manage it. It is my dream to have my own room.

As well as suboptimal living conditions, there are physical barriers in the form of checkpoints which prevent the free movement of Palestinian people on a daily basis, resulting in occupational deprivation. The accounts by all participants of the experience of the checkpoints related not just to the negative impacts of the amount of time spent at them daily, but the fear generated at the checkpoints with respect to demeanour and presentation. As one participant below says, we have to *be our best self* for fear of potentially being shot:

> The main challenge is waiting at the checkpoints, the queue because they want to check us ... I was lucky to get permission to work but the check points used to take 3 hours from me, it was so tiring I started to look for other jobs because it was tough. I found work in Hebron and one day we waited for hours, and it was risky, it's a road where a lot of Palestinians have been shot.
>
> The biggest single barrier is the check point, we have to be our best self, avoid eye contact. The problem in cars is if they don't see you they may shoot. I try to be polite but it's humiliating when a 16 year old is screaming at you and your mum to get back in line.

Groups lead to trouble: culture of surveillance and reprisals

As well as physical (and political/legislative) barriers, participants reflected on a perceived culture of surveillance, in which their actions (however seemingly innocuous to them) are noted and for which they will experience a reprisal in the form of an implicit or explicit threat, exclusion or possibly incarceration. Public or group forms of occupational participation are considered particularly risky.

> Sometimes when going to university they will suddenly set up a checkpoint – I have missed classes and exams because of that – the stress can be too much, it puts such a load on young people that they don't want to participate. Last month there was a marathon [for freedom] but my mother said "no way" it's a black mark, they will come at night and ask why you did it. So, we are not free to move, or to do anything.
>
> As a young person there are a lot of activities I would like to do, for example, the dabka, it is a traditional Palestinian dance but like everything it has become linked to politics ... the dance is linked to how people used to work on the land, and we have lost the land, dancing [therefore] keeps the past but they don't want that. You can't be in the scouts, you get asked lots of questions for playing music. Groups lead to trouble, any group ...

Proposition 2: Occupational responses to oppressive/limiting conditions/ contexts are not homogeneous but rather reflect the knowledge (epistemic) constructions, life stage, and sociocultural identities of persons in those contexts.

Existence is resistance: doing non-violent resistance in different ways

Participants described diverse, heterogeneous ways of enacting non-violent resistance on a daily basis. These diverse ways of doing non-violent resistance reflect the ways of knowing – or epistemological constructions – of the participants as well as their life stage, gender, and occupational status. Accordingly, they reflect differing levels of agentic response.

> Every year the Ministry of sport do a Marathon, we ran for Palestine, we ran for freedom [and I felt] proud, especially as we had people with disabilities in the marathon, we also ran for prisoners, we ran for people in jail for their political belief.

Whilst the above story is about participating in the marathon as a form of agentic, non-violent resistance, the next two narrative extracts reflect the very different epistemological positions, with respect to boycotting Israeli goods. One knows that it is a form of non-violent resistance and enacts it, whilst the other "can't even think about it":

> I support the Arab economy by buying food only from them, not Israeli, clothes as well as food, everything.
> I buy Israeli products, I know many don't, but I don't think about it, I don't do it, I can't even think about it.

Maybe it's just too hard and overwhelming in the context in which a lot of everyday life and forms of occupational participation are so very difficult. Below, the narrative extracts include humour, selectively choosing non-violent protests, and educating future generations – all as forms of situated non-violent resistance:

> I once asked a student "why are you coming late to class all the time?" and he said "I've been at a striptease party at the checkpoint" and I said "what?" and he said "yes, I had to take off my shirt and shoes" – and then he decided to show us. He made a video about his daily trip to the university from his home, it was a good way for the class to reflect on what happens to him on a daily basis. He has to queue and has guns

pointed at him. I like that he is not being passive, not a victim but showing others what happens to him. It's a sign of resilience that he makes a joke and that he speaks openly about it. The difficulties are told through humour and jokes ...

I demonstrate and take my children to demonstrate because they need to know that how we live is not normal. I only attend peaceful, non-violent protests.

It's important to help our students – to think differently and positively – to take action, they can volunteer and help the community rebuilding after they receive their education – we can influence others to build a different community, or to help with the damage after all these years of occupation. That's why education is the main way of non-violent resistance.

Summary and conclusions

In this chapter we have presented some of the narrative data of persons living in Palestine in an attempt to further our understandings of how people respond occupationally, on a daily basis, to situations and contexts which are extreme and/or oppressive. They are, in essence, contexts in which occupational deprivation is endemic. Relative to the narrative data, we have presented two of three theoretical propositions generated from a preliminary analysis; the third will be discussed in future publications.

Being and doing in contexts in which basic rights – such as rights of freedom of movement or speech – are denied, seems grindingly difficult from the accounts reflected in this chapter. It is also evident that these restrictions result in an experience of occupational deprivation on a daily basis. Moreover, because of the oppressive context and difficulties associated with communication and representation, it is difficult for these realities to be represented justly. Accordingly, we – as the authors – have attempted to provide a voice for those living under these restrictive conditions and, through this, attempt to illuminate otherwise poorly understood, yet highly complex, occupational phenomena. It marks only the beginning of what we believe will be a scholarly project which will develop greater theoretical depth over time.

References

Durocher, E., Gibson, B.E., & Rappolt, S. (2014). Occupational justice: A conceptual review. *Journal of Occupational Science, 21*(4), pp. 418–430. doi:10.1080/14427 591.2013.775692.

Fricker, M. (2007). *Epistemic injustice: Power and the ethics of knowing.* Oxford: Oxford University Press.

Hocking, C. (2012). Occupation through the looking glass: Reflecting on occupational scientists' ontological assumptions. In G. Whiteford & C. Hocking (Eds.), *Occupational science: Society, inclusion, participation* (pp. 54–66). https://doi.org/10.1002/9781118281581.ch5.

Liamputtong, P. (2013). *Qualitative research methods.* Melbourne: Oxford University Press.

Molineux, M., & Whiteford, G. (in press). Occupational science: Genesis, evolution and future contribution. In E. Duncan (Ed.), *Foundations for practice in occupational therapy* (6th ed.). Edinburgh: Churchill Livingstone.

Ramugondo, E. (2015). Occupational consciousness. *Journal of Occupational Science,* 22(4), pp. 488–501. https://doi.org/10.1080/14427591.2015.1042516.

Whiteford, G., Jones, K., Rahal, C., & Suleman, A. (2018). The Participatory Occupational Justice Framework as a tool for change: Three contrasting case narratives. *Journal of Occupational Science,* 25(4), pp. 497–508. https://doi.org/10.1080/14427591.2018.1504607.

Part II

Researching the dark side of occupation

6 Homelessness and occupation

*Leonie Boland, Carrie Anne Marshall,
and Lee Ann Westover*

Background

Despite the wealth of high-income countries, homelessness is a global issue, with rates of homelessness continuing to rise across Europe (FEANSTA & Foundation Abbe Pierre, 2017), Canada (Gaetz, Dej, Richter, & Redman, 2016), the USA (Henry et al., 2018), New Zealand (Amore, 2016) and Australia (Australian Bureau of Statistics, 2018). These statistics do not include the numbers of persons who are refugees or displaced by conflict internationally. Regardless of national strategies to address the homelessness crisis, the overwhelming influence of poverty, unemployment, health, and wealth disparities, including a lack of housing affordability, has resulted in this shocking trend. As a consequence, people of all genders and ages are unnecessarily suffering in some of the highest-income countries in the world. Homelessness is not only the absence of secure and adequate housing, it is an extreme form of social exclusion and is intrinsically linked with ill health and premature mortality (Bharel, 2016; Fazel, Geddes, & Kushel, 2014).

The experience of being homeless impacts on all aspects of a person's life, the opportunities that are available, and the choices that one can make. An occupational perspective presents a unique and valuable viewpoint within homelessness research, as it places a focus on the everyday lives of people and helps illuminate the reality of how individuals spend their time. As a concept, what people do with their time is largely ignored within homelessness policy and research. For example, housing success following homelessness is predominantly measured in the number of days housed, not the quality or experience of this living (Boland, Slade, Yarwood, & Bannigan, 2018).

Homelessness is experienced within a socio-economic and political context, where the complex interplay of poverty, health inequities, unemployment, and other social injustices generates and restrict opportunities. The transactional perspective (Dickie, Cutchin, & Humphry, 2006) underpins this chapter reinforcing the "co-constitutive" nature of people and place when considering occupations within the context of homelessness. Furthermore, Rudman's (2010) construct of occupational possibilities provides a lens to focus attention on the more subtle assumptions and practices that shape occupations in the context of homelessness. Occupational possibilities are the everyday activities that people take for granted as what they can, and are expected to do. These occupations are created and supported by aspects of the wider system and, in turn, shape the structures and contexts in which people live (Rudman, 2010).

Over the past two decades, there has been a steady increase in occupational science and occupational therapy research related to persons experiencing homelessness. To fully understand the occupational experience of being homeless, attention must be paid to all occupations that provide meaning and purpose, as well as the assumptions and contexts that shape them. Everyday activities for people who are homeless can include begging/panhandling, collecting and selling items (e.g. bottles), sex work, and substance use, and yet these occupations are largely unexplored in research. Shedding light on this dark side of occupation within homelessness is necessary to inform service provision and practice. A recent comprehensive systematic review amalgamated the findings of this body of literature with studies from occupational therapy, occupational science, psychology, medicine, anthropology, sociology, and social work (Marshall, Boland, Westover, Wickett, et al., 2019). Thirteen studies and two dissertations, which represented at least n = 366 participants, were included to present the nature of occupational experiences for homeless persons. We draw upon findings from this systematic review, and other research, to illustrate the complexity of occupational experiences, opportunities, and possibilities for those who have experienced homelessness.

Factors that influence occupational possibilities for homeless persons

There are several forces that combine to determine the occupational lives of homeless persons, and influence their well-being. These include the social and institutional contexts in which homeless persons are situated. Restrictions on the occupations of this population can limit opportunities for social integration and belonging, as well as identity, meaning, and purpose.

Social contexts that restrict the time use of homeless persons

Several studies in occupational therapy and occupational science indicate that the structural contexts in which homeless persons spend their time, and the daily demands that they face in order to survive, severely restrict their engagement in activities of meaning (Marshall, Boland, Westover, Wickett, et al., 2019). Poverty, the need to engage in activities for survival, and the stigma of homelessness can all impose restrictions on the time use of homeless persons, resulting in often profound social and occupational exclusion that imposes deleterious impacts on health and well-being.

As homelessness is primarily an issue caused by poverty (Gaetz et al., 2016), this is a likely cause of exclusion from occupations for many homeless persons. Poverty can limit one's time use simply because one is unable to afford the resources or gain access to environments that cost money. Choices for engagement in activities of meaning, thus, become severely restricted (Marshall, Lysaght, & Krupa, 2017; Tryssenaar, Jones, & Lee, 1999).

The need to survive

The need to manage survival on a daily basis has been identified as a determinant of time use for homeless persons across several studies (Butchinsky, 2004; Cunningham & Slade, 2019; Illman, Spence, O'Campo, & Kirsh, 2013; Marshall et al., 2017). Engaging in occupations such as securing food, earning money through illicit or unconventional employment, and securing resources to manage in inclement weather are examples of survival occupations that are necessary for homeless persons to function in contexts with limited resources.

Stigma

In addition to the oppression of poverty and social exclusion, homelessness is known to be associated with serious social stigma, a phenomenon that is marked by the visibility of homeless persons in public spaces (Lee, Tyler, & Wright, 2010). The social exclusion that results is likely to seriously limit possibilities for engaging in occupations with others in society. Those experiencing homelessness frequently express the fear of stigma once their homelessness has ended: "I do have concerns about stigma ... Particularly, how long I've been homeless will be a hindrance to me finding employment, as I'll be recognized as that homeless guy on the street" [Star] (Marshall et al., 2017, p. 174).

Institutional influences

An overt consequence of homelessness is dependence on services to meet basic needs (e.g. shelter and food). Unsurprisingly, institutional processes – structure, rules and routines – of hostels/shelters and social services organisations determine the time use of homeless persons (Marshall, Boland et al., 2019). The imposed rules restrict the occupational lives of service users and result in many feeling trapped in the system of services meant to serve them (Chard, Faulkner, & Chugg, 2009; Cunningham & Slade, 2019; Schultz-Krohn, 2004; Tryssenaar et al., 1999). This sense of entrapment can impact on a person's sense of self, identity, and in turn may affect their process of leaving homelessness: "It's a homeless place but you get used to the place. I was getting stuck ... Will I survive on my own again?" [Bernice] (Boland, 2018, p. 167). This is amplified for those parenting children while being supported by shelter and other services, in that rules imposed by these services often diminish parental authority and lead to a loss of self-efficacy (Salsi et al., 2017; Schultz-Krohn, 2004).

Beyond immediate physical and social environments, the socio-economic and political context determines the housing, welfare, and employment institutions that people must access in their transition from homelessness. The impact of being forced to navigate these services often takes up a large portion of the day for homeless persons, creating a role as "human service consumers" (Marshall, Boland, Westover, Wickett, et al., 2019). It is paradoxical that the same supports and services that enable a person to leave homelessness also frequently fill their time with appointments, meetings, and therapeutic groups that limit engagement in occupations that provide purpose and a genuine connection with others (Bukowski & Buetow, 2011; Illman et al., 2013; Wagner, 1994). These concepts have been relatively unexplored, and are in need of study in future research.

Consequences of exclusion from occupations for homeless persons

The end result of having one's occupations restricted by poverty, the need to survive, stigma, and institutional factors is that homeless persons frequently report spending significant periods of time in which they are relatively unoccupied, or occupied in activities that hold little meaning for them (Marshall et al., 2017). Contrary to common perception, this situation does not improve once one becomes housed, and in some cases, these periods of unoccupied time become even more pronounced on leaving homelessness (Marshall, Lysaght, & Krupa, 2018). Boredom that is both severe and pervasive is frequently reported by homeless persons, and is associated with negative impacts on mental well-being (Marshall, Davidson, et al., 2019; Marshall, Roy et al., 2019). Furthermore, homeless persons who are both unoccupied and exposed in public are more likely to be victimised by others (Garland, Richards, & Cooney, 2010). These impacts on the well-being of homeless persons make an occupational perspective on homelessness a particularly important one for policy, practice, and research.

The critical importance of an occupational perspective

An occupational perspective reveals important possibilities for addressing the health and social inequities faced by those with lived experiences of homelessness. All humans thrive in environments that nurture engagement in occupation, as this enables us to gain a sense of meaning, purpose, identity, and the ability to connect with others. Existing research suggests that occupation shares an important relationship with key outcomes that can improve the lives of homeless persons, such as being integrated in one's community, mental well-being, and quality of life.

Occupation as a means of social integration and belonging

Co-occupation, or being involved in an activity with one or more persons (Pickens & Pizur-Barnekow, 2009), is one of the primary ways in which homeless persons connect with others, and form a sense of belonging. As many homeless persons lack opportunities to engage in activities that are meaningful to them, this can severely limit social integration and belonging in one's community. Interdisciplinary literature on homelessness indicates that poor community integration is a significant problem experienced by homeless persons before and after homelessness (Gaetz et al., 2016). In a recent systematic review of interventions for homeless persons that measured community integration as an outcome, few strategies improved social integration, belonging, and time spent in the broader community (Marshall, Boland, Westover, Marcellus, et al., 2019). Those that were identified to be effective in promoting community integration included occupational interventions such as supported employment and social enterprise, and those that linked participants directly with others, such as peer support and psychoeducation (Marshall, Boland, Westover, Marcellus, et al., 2019).

The occupations in which we engage alone or with others typically inform our sense of individual and collective identity. The experience of homelessness can exclude people from access to mainstream activities and bring them together in the context of public spaces (Wagner, 1994). In some studies, having an identity as a "street family" member is reported to be reinforced by engaging in activities with or for others on the street, for example cooking for one another (Bukowski & Buetow, 2011), or drinking (Radley, Hodgetts & Cullen, 2005). These street-based occupations strengthened relationships and facilitated belonging. The support derived from these natural social networks and social functioning contributes to resilience in homeless individuals (Durbin et al., 2019), and needs to be promoted in practice and policy aimed at supporting the health and well-being of this population.

Deriving meaning, purpose, and identity through occupation

The occupations in which we engage provide us with a sense of meaning in our lives, provide us with purpose and a sense of accomplishment, and help us to know who we are as individuals. Commonplace occupations taken for granted by housed persons can hold existential or spiritual significance, and lead to feelings of personal transformation. For instance, street homeless individuals who were given the opportunity to shower in one study (Cunningham & Slade, 2019, p. 23) described the experience with deep gratitude – as "priceless". In the context of engaging in occupation, participants in some studies experienced a sense of quiet that gave rise to both personal revelations (Chard et al., 2009; Iveson & Cornish, 2016; Tryssenaar et al., 1999), and a sense of order to an otherwise chaotic life (Salsi et al., 2017).

Occupation as a form of coping

Events which lead to homelessness such as relationship breakdowns, substance use, and unemployment, can be understood as profound life transitions which result in comprehensive changes in habits and routines. It follows that stress and anxiety precede and accompany this transition, and individuals use a wide range of occupations to cope with the unpredictability of a homeless life. The use of substances, which are widely available to homeless persons, is both a way of coping and something that often structures the time and identities of homeless persons (Bukowski & Buetow, 2011; Butchinsky, 2004; Marshall et al., 2017).

Conclusion

Within the context of homelessness, research has shown that engagement in occupations can provide a sense of meaning, purpose, and connection, which can positively influence health and well-being. This finding has implications for improving the lives of people who, as a result of homelessness, experience extreme social and health inequities. As occupational scientists and therapists we have an ethical obligation to bring the value of an occupational perspective to the fore at a policy and organisational level. This has the potential to influence homelessness service provision by shaping expectations and structures to provide opportunities for meaningful occupational engagement. To do this successfully, the dark side, or unacknowledged aspects, of the occupational lives of homeless persons must be uncovered. Extending a focus beyond occupations that are solely health-promoting may provide a challenge to occupational therapists but if occupation-based strategies to support people to transition from homelessness are to be realistic and effective, attention must be paid to their full range of occupations.

References

Amore, K. (2016). *Severe housing deprivation in Aotearoa/New Zealand: 2001–2013*. Wellington: He Kainga Oranga/Housing & Health Research Programme, University of Otago. Retrieved from www.healthyhousing.org.nz/wp-content/uploads/2016/08/Severe-housing-deprivation-in-Aotearoa-2001-2013-1.pdf.

Australian Bureau of Statistics (2018). Census of Population and Housing: Estimating homelessness, 2016, cat. no. 2049.0. Retrieved from www.abs.gov.au/AUSSTATS/abs@.nsf/allprimarymainfeatures/ED457E1CF56EA15ECA257A7500148DB3?op endocument.

Bharel, M. (2016). Emergency care for homeless patients: A window into the health needs of vulnerable populations. *American Journal of Public Health, 106*(5), pp. 784–785. doi:10.2105/AJPH.2016.303161.

Boland, L. (2018). Transitioning from homelessness into a sustained tenancy: What enables successful tenancy sustainment? (The Moving on Project) (Doctoral Dissertation, University of Plymouth, Plymouth, UK). Retrieved from https://pearl.plymouth.ac.uk/handle/10026.1/11660.

Boland, L., Slade, A., Yarwood, R., & Bannigan, K. (2018). Determinants of tenancy sustainment following homelessness: A systematic review. *American Journal of Public Health, 108*(11), e1–e8. doi:10.2105/AJPH.2018.304652.

Bukowski, K., & Buetow, S. (2011). Making the invisible visible: A Photovoice exploration of homeless women's health and lives in central Auckland. *Social Science Medicine, 72*(5), pp. 739–746.

Butchinsky, C. (2004). An anthropological study of repeated homelessness in Oxford. Retrieved from https://ethos.bl.uk/OrderDetails.do?uin=uk.bl.ethos.404751.

Chard, G., Faulkner, T., & Chugg, A. (2009). Exploring occupation and its meaning among homeless men. *British Journal of Occupational Therapy, 72*(3), pp. 116–124.

Cunningham, M.J., & Slade, A. (2019). Exploring the lived experience of homelessness from an occupational perspective. *Scandinavian Journal of Occupational Therapy, 26*(1), pp. 19–32. doi:10.1080/11038128.2017.1304572.

Dickie, V., Cutchin, M.P., & Humphry, R. (2006). Occupation as transactional experience: A critique of individualism in occupational science. *Journal of Occupational Science, 13*(1), pp. 83–93.

Durbin, A., Nisenbaum, R., Kopp, B., O'Campo, P., Hwang, S.W., & Stergiopoulos, V. (2019). Are resilience and perceived stress related to social support and housing stability among homeless adults with mental illness? *Health & Social Care in the Community, 27*(4), pp. 1053–1062. doi:10.1111/hsc.12722.

Fazel, S., Geddes, J.R., & Kushel, M. (2014). The health of homeless people in high-income countries: Descriptive epidemiology, health consequences, and clinical and policy recommendations. *The Lancet, 384*(9953), pp. 1529–1540. doi:10.1016/S0140-6736(14)61132-6.

FEANSTA & Foundation Abbe Pierre (2017). Second overview of housing exclusion in Europe 2017. Retrieved from www.feantsa.org/download/gb_housing-exclusion-report_complete_20178613899107250251219.pdf.

Gaetz, S., Dej, E., Richter, T., & Redman, M. (2016). The state of homelessness in Canada 2016. Retrieved from http://homelesshub.ca/sites/default/files/SOHC16_final_20Oct2016.pdf.

Garland, T.S., Richards, T., & Cooney, M. (2010). Victims hidden in plain sight: The reality of victimization among the homeless. *Criminal Justice Studies, 23*(4), pp. 285–301. doi:10.1080/1478601X.2010.516525.

Henry, M., Mahathey, A., Morrill, T., Robinson, A., Shivji, A., & Watt, R. (2018). The 2018 Annual Homeless Assessment Report (AHAR) to Congress. Retrieved from https://files.hudexchange.info/resources/documents/2018-AHAR-Part-1.pdf.

Illman, S.C., Spence, S., O'Campo, P.J., & Kirsh, B.H. (2013). Exploring the occupations of homeless adults living with mental illnesses in Toronto. *Canadian Journal of Occupational Therapy*, 80(4), pp. 215–223. doi:10.1177/0008417413 506555.

Iveson, M., & Cornish, F. (2016). Re-building bridges: Homeless people's views on the role of vocational and educational activities in their everyday lives. *Journal of Community & Applied Social Psychology*, 26(3), pp. 253–267. https://doi.org/10. 1002/casp.2262.

Lee, B.A., Tyler, K.A., & Wright, J.D. (2010). The new homelessness revisited. *Annual Review of Sociology*, 36, pp. 501–521. doi:10.1146/annurev-soc-z070 308-115940.

Marshall, C.A., Boland, L., Westover, L., Marcellus, B., Weil, S., Meaney, H., & Wickett, S. (2019). Community integration interventions for homeless persons: A systematic review. Manuscript in development.

Marshall, C.A., Boland, L., Westover, L.A., Wickett, S., Roy, L., Gewurtz, R.E., ... Kirsh, B. (2019). Occupational experiences of homeless persons: A systematic review and meta-aggregation. Manuscript submitted for publication.

Marshall, C.A., Davidson, L., Li, A., Gewurtz, R., Roy, L., Barbic, S., ... Lysaght, R. (2019). Boredom and meaningful activity in adults experiencing homelessness: A mixed-methods study. *Canadian Journal of Occupational Therapy*, 86(5), pp. 357–370. doi:10.1177/0008417419833402.

Marshall, C.A., Lysaght, R., & Krupa, T. (2017). The experience of occupational engagement of chronically homeless persons in a mid-sized urban context. *Journal of Occupational Science*, 24(2), pp. 165–180. doi:10.1080/14427591.2016.1277548.

Marshall, C.A., Lysaght, R., & Krupa, T. (2018). Occupational transition in the process of becoming housed following chronic homelessness. *Canadian Journal of Occupational Therapy*, 85(1), pp. 33–45. doi:10.1177/0008417417723351.

Marshall, C.A., Roy, L., Becker, A., Nguyen, M., Barbic, S., Tjörnstrand, C., ... Wickett, S. (2019). Boredom and homelessness: A scoping review. *Journal of Occupational Science*, 27(1), pp. 107–124. doi:10.1080/14427591.2019.1595095.

Pickens, N.D., & Pizur-Barnekow, K. (2009). Co-occupation: Extending the dialogue. *Journal of Occupational Science*, 16(3), pp. 151–156. doi:10.1080/14427591.2 009.9686656.

Radley, A., Hodgetts, D., & Cullen, A. (2005). Visualizing homelessness: A study in photography and estrangement. *Journal of Community & Applied Social Psychology*, 15(4), pp. 273–295. doi:10.1002/casp.825.

Rudman, D.L. (2010). Occupational terminology: Occupational possibilities. *Journal of Occupational Science*, 17(1), pp. 55–59.

Salsi, S., Awadallah, Y., Leclair, A.B., Breault, M.-L., Duong, D.-T., & Roy, L. (2017). Occupational needs and priorities of women experiencing homelessness. *Canadian Journal of Occupational Therapy*, 84(4–5), pp. 229–241. doi:10.1177/ 0008417417719725.

Schultz-Krohn, W. (2004). The meaning of family routines in a homeless shelter. *American Journal of Occupational Therapy*, 58(5), pp. 531–542.

Tryssenaar, J., Jones, E.J., & Lee, D. (1999). Occupational performance needs of a shelter population. *Canadian Journal of Occupational Therapy*, 66(4), pp. 188–196. doi:10.1177/000841749906600406.

Wagner, D. (1994). Beyond the pathologizing of nonwork: Alternative activities in a street community. *Social Work*, 39(6), pp. 718–727.

7 Occupational transition from smoker to non-smoker

The perceived consequences in women's lives

Kerrie Luck

Introduction

Smoking tobacco is a substantial threat to the health of our population. It is the world's leading preventable cause of death and disease, killing more than seven million people annually (WHO, 2017). Unfortunately, occupations, such as smoking, that are commonly regarded as "unhealthy" and addictive, are not as readily represented in the occupational science or occupational therapy literature (Kiepek, Beagan, Lalibert Rudman & Phelan, 2019; Twinley, 2013). This limited view restricts our understanding of how the multiple facets of this occupation impact well-being (Twinley & Addidle, 2012; Twinley, 2013), and construct value, meaning, identity and purpose in one's life (Luck, 2013). While the majority of individuals who smoke report they want to quit, it may take over 30 quit attempts before quitting for good (Chaiton et al., 2016). Exploring the transition of smoker[1] to non-smoker from an occupational perspective offers insight into the factors that may influence smoking, smoking cessation, and relapse rates (Luck & Beagan, 2015). Authorities suggest even small improvements in smoking cessation success rates could have a significant effect on tobacco use prevalence and the overall health of the population (WHO, 2017). Through conducting this study,[2] I sought to gain a greater understanding of how the occupational transition, from smoker to non-smoker, was experienced and perceived.

While smoking is often viewed by society as a "bad habit", experts confirm smoking is an addiction to nicotine with many influential factors (i.e. biological, psychological, behavioural, cultural) that make it difficult to stop using tobacco, despite the harmful consequences (ASAM, 2013). These factors contribute to chronic relapse and the multiple quit attempts seen during the transition to a non-smoker (Chaiton et al., 2016). Helbig and McKay (2013) suggest many aspects of addiction can be occupational in nature, such as the use of time, routines, or day-to-day choices. The inherent recurrence of relapse suggests occupations aligned with new roles, opportunity for self-discovery, and meaningful use of time will support the transition process. Evidently, exploring individuals with addiction from an occupational perspective can facilitate exploration into the complex relationship between occupation and addictions – thus allowing for "occupation to be utilized as a means to maximize health, human capacities, and as an approach to breaking the cycle of addiction" (Helbig & McKay, 2013, p. 144).

Occupational transitions and loss

Occupational transitions are common in our everyday life and can include various aspects of loss, adaptation, and identity formation (Luck & Beagan, 2015). They occur when there is a shift from one occupation to another and can be self-initiated, part of a developmental process, or due to a life event (Townsend & Polatajko, 2007). In the case of smoking cessation, the transition from smoker to non-smoker can be initiated for a multitude of reasons, such as the drive to alleviate the social stigma of smoking, pressure from a loved one, a desire for a healthier lifestyle, or in response to a medical condition (Salive et al., 1992). Often smokers underestimate the impact of quitting; the inability to engage in familiar occupations associated with smoking may not only contribute to a feeling of loss and distress but also affect identity and self-esteem (Blair, 2000). The degree to which this is experienced depends on the level of importance and meaning the occupation held (Townsend & Polatajko, 2007).

Occupational identity and adaptation

The reciprocal reliance between the occupations we do and how we view ourselves when doing them, contributes to our occupational identity. Inversely our sense of self also drives the occupations we engage in (Laliberte Rudman, 2002). Often, during a transition, a person's inability to engage in meaningful occupations can have an impact on their identity, especially if the changes are unforeseen, numerous, or involuntary (Vrkljan & Polgar, 2007). Collins, Maguire and O'Dell (2002) found smoking-related occupations facilitated social companionship, improved performance in unfamiliar social situations, and helped smokers "protect, project and maintain identity" (p. 649). As people adapt to changes in occupations during smoking cessation, they may redefine their sense of self (Vrkljan & Polgar, 2007).

To successfully manoeuvre a transition, people may change roles and find a balance of meaningful and valued occupations in order to maintain occupational performance (Blair, 2000). Occupational adaptation can enable an individual who has quit smoking to change what they do to respond to their environment when faced with challenges. Navigating the transition to non-smoker requires awareness and acknowledgement of the transition, and the ability to develop behaviours and occupations to deal with change (Blair, 2000). Seemingly, occupational performance is impacted when smokers do not foresee, or plan for, adjustments needed during the transition process (Vrkljan & Polgar, 2007).

Methods

The methodology that guided this study was interpretative phenomenological analysis (IPA), a qualitative methodology that examines how people make sense of their life experiences (Smith, Flowers, & Larkin, 2009). The sample was chosen through purposeful homogeneous sampling and consisted of seven women between the ages of 35 to 55, who self-reported having quit smoking at least 12 months, but no longer than 24 months, previously, and were still not smoking. Data were collected through in-depth, face-to-face, audio-recorded interviews that lasted between 60 and 90 minutes.

Findings

Twenty subthemes were identified; these were clustered into five superordinate themes which represent the participants' individualised accounts of their experiences and the researcher's interpretations. Themes and subthemes were developed using direct quotes from the participants (in vivo) to enhance credibility for the reader. Across each theme, varying dimensions of meaning, loss, occupational identity, and/or occupational adaptation were described. While all themes are displayed in Figure 7.1, only superordinate themes are described, with extracted quotes from the various subthemes, to illustrate the richness of the findings.

Let's go ... have a smoke

This theme provides a foundation to understand the lived experiences as a smoker. It illustrates how smoking was a meaningful, prioritised occupation that fostered structure in their daily life, a sense of belonging, and social connectiveness. Conversely, a lack of control over smoking and relapse contributed to a sense of failure, secrecy, and shame.

> When you're a smoker, everything revolves around the next cigarette, so you [use it to] measure time.
>
> ("Donna")

> We had something in common ... was something that we did together.
>
> ("Betty")

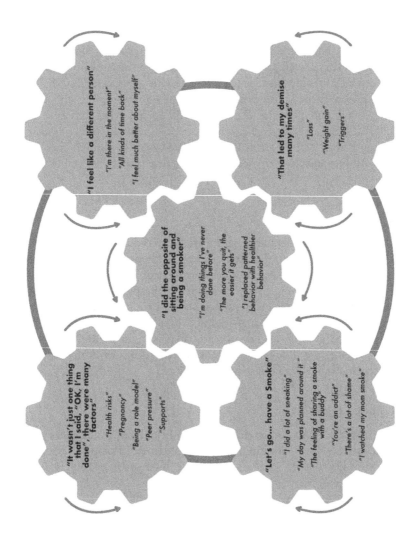

Figure 7.1 The occupational transition from smoking to non-smoking.

Hiding stuff and being sneaky all the time, it's very stressful, it's just very stressful and very degrading, being a sneaky person sucks.

("Greta") (Luck & Beagan, 2015, p. 189)

It wasn't just one thing that I said, "OK, I'm done", there were many factors

There were many motivations and supports that helped the women to progress throughout the occupational transition to a non-smoker, as well as getting back on the path of trying to quit after relapse. For instance, supports included: medication, help-lines, friends and family, hypnosis, and seeing others quit. No clear motivator or support was principally responsible; rather, it appeared to be a combination of many factors that created a suitable environment for their own transition. Peer pressure, social stigma, and smoke-free legislation challenged their self-worth and occupational identity, while at the same time influenced their changing behaviours and occupations. Consequently, they felt they became a non-smoker, and a role model for others.

When you get negative feedback from non-smokers ... all I would see is how I really viewed myself reflected in them.

(Donna)

I guess that's the thing, trying to be a role model for your kids and showing them.

(Betty)

That led to my demise many times

Many barriers were experienced during the occupational transition to non-smoker. Occupational loss was a significant obstacle experienced when knowingly giving up or adapting an occupation that triggered smoking behaviour, or when it was linked directly to smoking itself, such as using smoking as a mechanism for coping, concentration, an incentive, or "me" time. These not only created challenges to successful adaptation, but also contributed to previous unsuccessful quit attempts.

You lose your best friend, because it was always there for you ... it doesn't matter, three in the morning, you can't sleep, it's there.

(Betty)

You would reward yourself, if I get that done ... or if I get this done ... then I can sit outside and I can have a cigarette.

(Betty) (Luck & Beagan, 2015, p. 189)

I did the opposite of sitting around and being a smoker

A change in doing and adapting of occupations assisted in maintaining participation in activities that created meaning and purpose, which in turn allowed the women to "*re-invent*" themselves as non-smokers and supported their new occupational identity. Quitting smoking was not a single occurrence for any of the women, it was a meaningful, ongoing, and valued occupational experience that allowed them to gain insights, build skills and occupational competence in their transition to a non-smoker.

> You kinda have to re-invent yourself, so I'm doing things that I never did before, I'm gardening for the first time in my life.
>
> (Greta)

> Each time I quit smoking I learned something that helped me … you're restructuring how you do things on a day-to-day basis, minute-to-minute, your association with friends, with food, with activities, with time, everything is completely shifted and there is no way a person can learn that in one fell swoop … You're practicing quitting each time you do it.
>
> (Donna) (Luck & Beagan, 2015, pp. 190–191)

I feel like a different person

The vivid illustrations provided by the participants paint a powerful picture of how the occupational transition to becoming and being a non-smoker has impacted their lives; from strengthening relationships, improving self-esteem and feelings of accomplishment, to having more time to engage in other meaningful and valued occupations as a non-smoker. The favourable experiences and perceptions of being a non-smoker nurtured a positive occupational identity that reinforced their successful occupational transition.

> I'm there for them and I'm not preoccupied … to be there and just to listen, not have to worry about going anywhere.
>
> (Betty)

> The biggest thing I think I've gained by quitting is liking myself more.
>
> (Greta)

Discussion

These findings demonstrate smoking was a valued and meaningful occupation to women trying to quit. It was also associated with varying consequences for each woman's daily subjective experience of health, well-being, and occupation. In order to accurately understand the multiple facets of this transition, it is essential to challenge assumptions made about smoking as an occupation. Occupation-focused practice must fully embrace and appreciate an individual's occupational life, including occupations that may not traditionally be viewed as positive, productive, or healthy (Twinley, 2013), so as to ensure an accurate understanding of what people do in their daily lives (Kiepek et al., 2019). Exploring experiences of addiction-as-occupation may uncover factors impeding recovery, as well as informing future research and intervention practice (Wasmuth, Crabtree, & Scott, 2014). Similar to research conducted by Creek and Hughes (2008), this study showed health benefits and risks were not always "mutually exclusive" (p. 464). Townsend and Polatajko (2007) endorse this point, stating, "The idiosyncrasy of occupations point to an important caveat. Not all occupations lead to health, wellbeing and justice or have therapeutic value, even if they hold meaning, organize time and bring structure to life" (p. 22).

The occupational identity attached to smoking was twofold: positive and meaningful in relation to other smokers – an identity of connection, belonging, and structure; yet, also negative in relation to others (often nonsmokers) in society – an identity of shame, secrecy, and guilt. In the case of tobacco, social norms have been shown to influence how individuals feel about themselves, as well as their intentions to quit and ability to stay quit (Betzner et al., 2012). The conflict of social perceptions and feelings of loss described by the women not only challenged their occupational identity, but also the transition process itself. Similarly, this was seen by Seguire and Chalmers (2000), where women quit smoking and relapsed based on the meaning smoking held in their lives; referring to it as the "cost of quitting" (p. 227). During their transition, the women in my study engaged in new occupations, viewed by themselves and others as "healthy" (within a sociocultural context identified as Western and largely individualistic), not only to replace smoking-related occupations, but also to foster a non-smoker identity. The transitions back-and-forth from smoker to non-smoker allowed the women to practise, adapt to changes, gain insights, and build occupational competence in the skills needed to transition successfully to their goal of being a non-smoker.

Implications for occupational therapy practice

My findings validate the complexity of smoking cessation transitions and the important role all occupations play. This revealed important implications for occupational therapy.

First, a broader view of what the occupation of smoking entails should be sought to enhance understanding of how smoking can contribute to well-being. This would include acknowledging the role and meaning smoking plays in people's daily lives. Here, I am mindful of Twinley and Morris' (2014, p. 275) caution that this may "involve working in a way that makes us feel uncomfortable, and that presents us with ethical, legal, and moral dilemmas".

Second, enabling individuals to participate in meaningful occupations that support their aim to transition to a non-smoker can provide a sense of purpose and structure, as well as nurture occupational identity, ultimately supporting overall occupational performance.

Third, education on the cyclical nature of relapse, viewing it as an opportunity to practise and adapt new occupations (versus a failure to transition), is an important part of enabling. Also, encouraging reflection and coaching skill development and adaptation to build occupational competence in order to meet the demands of the environment is also imperative.

Occupational therapists are uniquely equipped to enable clients to engage in everyday living through the use of occupation. This expertise can be utilised within smoking cessation and relapse prevention. As an occupational therapist, researcher, and certified tobacco educator, it is my hope these findings expand our concept of what constitutes an occupation, in addition to highlighting the complex relationship between health, well-being, and all occupations.

Notes

1 While the author prefers to refer to the participants as "individuals who smoke", the participants described and referred to themselves as a "smoker"; hence, this is the term used throughout.
2 Additional details can be found at https://dalspace.library.dal.ca/handle/10222/21440. Parts of this study have also been published in the *Journal of Occupational Science* (Luck & Beagan, 2015).

References

ASAM: American Society of Addiction Medicine (2013). Definition of addiction. Retrieved from www.asam.org/for-the-public/definition-of-addiction.

Betzner, A.E., Boyle, R.G., Luxenberg, M.G., Schillo, B.A., Keller, P.A., Rainey, J., ... Saul, J.E. (2012). Experience of smokers and recent quitters with smoke-free regulations and quitting. *American Journal of Preventative Medicine, 43*(5S3), S163–S170.

Blair, S.E. (2000). The centrality of occupation during life transitions. *British Journal of Occupational Therapy, 63*(5), pp. 231–237.

Chaiton, M., Diemert, L., Cohen, J.E., Bondy, S. J., Selby, P., Philipneri, A., & Schwartz. R. (2016). Estimating the number of quit attempts it takes to quit smoking successfully in a longitudinal cohort of smokers. *BMJ Open, 6*(6), pp. 1–9. doi:10.1136/bmjopen-2016-011045.

Collins, P., Maguire, M., & O'Dell, L. (2002). Smokers' representations of their own smoking: A q-methodological study. *Journal of Health Psychology, 7*(6), pp. 641–652. doi:10.1177/1359105302007006868.

Creek, J., & Hughes, A. (2008). Occupation and health: A review of selected literature. *British Journal of Occupational Therapy, 71*(11), pp. 456–468.

Helbig, K., & McKay, E. (2003). An exploration of addictive behaviours from an occupational perspective. *Journal of Occupational Science, 10*(3), pp. 140–145.

Kiepek, N.C., Beagan, B., Laliberte Rudman, D., & Phelan, S. (2019). Silences around occupations framed as unhealthy, illegal, and deviant. *Journal of Occupational Science, 26*(3), pp. 341–353. doi:10.1080/14427591.2018.1499123.

Laliberte Rudman, D. (2002) Linking occupation and identity: Lessons learned through qualitative exploration. *Journal of Occupational Science*, 9(1), pp. 12–19.

Luck, K.E. (2013). Occupational transition of smoking cessation in women: More than just butting out (Master's thesis, Dalhousie University, Halifax, Nova Scotia). Retrieved from https://dalspace.library.dal.ca/bitstream/handle/10222/21440/Luck-Kerrie-MSc-OTPP-May-2013.pdf?sequence=1&isAllowed=y.

Luck, K., & Beagan, B. (2015). Occupational transition of smoking cessation in women: "You're restructuring your whole life". *Journal of Occupational Science*, 22(2), pp. 183–196. doi:10.1080/14427591.2014.887418.

Pierce, D. (2001). Untangling occupation and activity. *The American Journal of Occupational Therapy*, 55(2), pp. 138–146.

Salive, M.E., Cornoni-Huntley, J., LaCroix, A.Z., Ostfeld, A.M., Wallace, R.B., & Hennekens, C.H. (1992). Predictors of smoking cessation and relapse in older adults. *American Journal of Public Health*, 82(9), pp. 1268–1271.

Seguire, M., & Chalmers, K. (2000). Addressing the "costs of quitting smoking": A health promotion issue for adolescent girls in Canada. *Health Promotion International*, 15(3), pp. 227–235.

Smith, J.A., Flowers, P., & Larkin, M. (2009). *Interpretative Phenomenological Analysis: Theory, method and research*. London: Sage Publications.

Townsend, E., & Polatajko, H. (2007). *Enabling occupation II: Advancing occupational therapy vision for health, well-being and justice through occupation*. Ottawa: CAOT Publications ACE.

Twinley, R. (2013). The dark side of occupation: A concept for consideration. *Australian Occupational Therapy Journal*, 60(4), pp. 301–303. doi:10.1111/1440-1630.12026.

Twinley, R., & Addidle, G. (2012). Considering violence: The dark side of occupation. *British Journal of Occupational Therapy*, 75(4), pp. 202–204. doi:10.4276/0308 02212X13336366278257.

Twinley, R., & Morris, K. (2014). Are we achieving occupation-focused practice? *British Journal of Occupational Therapy*, 77(6), p. 275. https://doi.org/10.4276/0308 02214X14018723137922.

Vrkljan, B.H., & Miller Polgar, J. (2007). Linking occupational participation and occupational identity: An exploratory study of the transition from driving to driving cessation in older adulthood. *Journal of Occupational Science*, 14(1), pp. 30–39. doi:10.1080/14427591.2007.9686581.

Wasmuth, S., Crabtree, J.L., & Scott, P.J. (2014). Exploring addiction-as-occupation. *British Journal of Occupational Therapy*, 77(12), pp. 605–613. doi:10.4276/030 802214X14176260335264.

World Health Organization (WHO) (2017). WHO report on the global tobacco epidemic, 2017: Monitoring tobacco use and prevention policies. Retrieved from www.who.int/tobacco/global_report/2017/en/.

8 Self-defeating behaviour in an individual with borderline personality disorder from an occupational perspective

Sarah Mercer

Introduction

In this chapter, I aim to present the concept of "self-defeating occupations" as experienced within the context of conditions such as Borderline Personality Disorder (BPD) or Complex Post Traumatic Stress Disorder (Complex PTSD). The origins of considering the dark side of occupations embedded within self-harm and eating disorders, which are commonly associated with these conditions, are presented, followed by a deeper exploration of "Emily's" experience.

Concept

My interest in self-defeating behaviours from an occupational perspective originated from personal experience. For many years my time was absorbed by self-harm and eating disorders to such a level that I had multiple involuntary hospital admissions. At the time I could not imagine a life that was not dominated by self-harm and all the rituals and activities contained within an eating disorder. Recovery seemed like a bleak and empty prospect. Part of the problem was that when I engaged in treatment, although the self-harm would be acknowledged by therapists (both psychotherapeutic and occupational), it felt like discussing it in any depth was taboo. This had the result of feeling that a large part of my experience was lost and poorly understood, but primarily that those occupations that were sustaining me were 'wrong' or 'bad', which only added to my emotional distress.

While my recovery was far from straightforward and involved the synthesis of many types of therapy, a large part of it occurred once I worked with an occupational therapist who was comfortable with deep occupational analysis of those rarely considered occupations. This piqued my interest in occupational therapy as a career and it was during my under-graduate studies that I was able to reflect on my own experiences from an occupational science standpoint. With support from tutors I began to write a blog examining the concept of "self-defeating occupation", and from this developed a research proposal to further explore the construct.

Definitions

I consider self-defeating behaviour (SDB) as "any deliberate or intentional behaviour that has clear, definitely or probably negative effects on the self or on the self's projects" (Baumeister & Scher, 1988, p. 3). While self-defeating behaviour is common within non-clinical populations (Baumeister & Scher, 1988), the use of behaviour that fits the definition has long been associated with people diagnosed with BPD (Gallop, 1992). I intended to examine common behaviours, such as cutting, burning, and eating disordered behaviours, but used the definition to avoid limitation and allow for self-assessment of what may be self-defeating for an individual. Conducting this phenomenological study has led me to assert the need to consider SDB as occupation. Due to minimal consideration of the dark side of occupations – such as self-harm and eating disorders – within the literature, the term "behaviour" was used to examine the existing knowledge-base.

Similarly, the diagnosis of BPD is a controversial one, with emerging consideration of the experiences of people with the condition better attributed to Complex PTSD. I used the more established construct "BPD" to frame the population of interest, with awareness there may be parallels with people with other diagnoses, such as Emotionally Unstable Personality Disorder or Complex PTSD.

Existing concepts

At the time of conducting the research there was emerging consideration of the dark side of occupations, such as those related to violence (Twinley & Addidle, 2012), and addiction (Wasmuth, Crabtree, & Scott, 2014). While not examined in the case of people diagnosed with BPD, Elliot (2012) provided an occupational perspective on eating disorders. Within the field of BPD, self-defeating behaviour research had focused on physiological or psychological functions of the behaviours. These concepts, combined with personal understanding, prompted an exploratory study which aimed to examine the meaning of self-defeating behaviour for an individual with BPD from an occupational perspective.

The research

The complexity of the experience of engaging in self-defeating occupations is suited to a phenomenological study that explores the personal understanding of such an experience (Denscombe, 2010), and is particularly applicable to a subject not yet considered in the literature (Polit & Beck, 2012). Full ethical approval was granted by the University Health Subjects' Research Ethics Committee. Subsequently, I conducted a single case study (Emily) as a method to generate detailed and complex data, and as an initial study in this area (Baxter & Jack, 2008). Since the aim of the study required meaning-making of the phenomenon of self-defeating occupations for Emily – which occurred through my interpretation of Emily's meaning-making, and was assisted by my own experience – a double hermeneutic occurred (Palmer, 1969). This position lends the data to analysis by Interpretative Phenomenological Analysis (IPA) (Smith, Flowers, & Larkin, 2010), as a method of capturing the double hermeneutic (Smith, 2004). Hermeneutics is the "practice or art of interpretation" (Dallmayr, 2009, p. 23) and the require-ment for a double hermeneutic is to interpret how "the participant is trying to make sense of their personal and social world; [and] the researcher is trying to make sense of the participant trying to make sense of their per-sonal and social world" (Smith, 2004, p. 40). The interview was semi-structured, allowing open-ended and probing questions to elicit the level of detail required (DePoy & Gitlin, 2011).

Findings

The findings illuminate the experience and meaning of SDB for Emily. Emily's understanding of SDB included various methods of self-harm (including personal use of self-cutting/burning/bleaching, overdosing with medication, and alcohol abuse), eating-disordered behaviour, attempting suicide, and less overt behaviour that conflicted with personal goals, such as not attending work. Her exploration of using SDB and engagement with mental health services was analysed, as illustrated in Figure 8.1, which situ-ates the subthemes within their respective superordinate theme.

"It's just all-consuming"

During Emily's interview it became apparent that while she identified engaging in SDB since the age of 8, there was a point in her mid-twenties where there was a notable increase in her use of SDB, at a time where "it all collapsed". Emily then explained how things deteriorated: "it was either waiting to die, or trying to die, or going into hospital, or out of hospital, it just was all-consuming, was self-harming".

The effect of engagement in such an all-encompassing occupation is likely to have reflected on Emily's identity; her reflection on the time cer-tainly allows understanding of someone who "was a day-to-day psychiatric patient". Moreover, her experience of increased use of SDB is one of it changing her identity to someone who "didn't do anything that was particu-larly me anymore", while the actual SDB "became my thing". Seemingly,

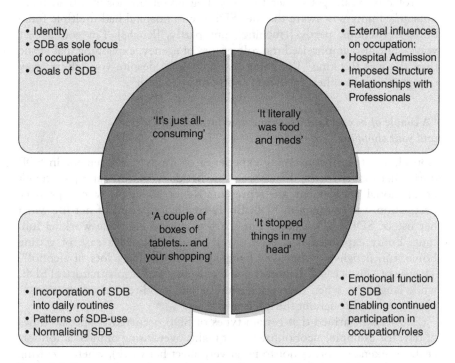

Figure 8.1 Superordinate themes (centre) and connected subthemes (outer).

Emily's experience of loss of occupational identity (such as being someone who was a "good" worker) was discussed as both causing and remedying her escalated use of SDB.

Insights as to why SDB was such an all-consuming occupation for Emily derive from her explanation of the over-arching goal of the SDB. Emily explained that she was not able to understand the precise reason for using SDB at the time, but that subsequent reflection confirms that it "gave me something to do that was destructive, that I wasn't already doing before".

"It literally was food and meds"

Much of this theme encompassed content relating to the effect of hospital admission on all occupational routines and engagement. There were specific consequences for the experience of SDB during hospital admission. Emily's experience of a daily routine in hospital was that her "pattern of day was dictated by theirs, and there wasn't anything to do". When asked if she continued to use SDB in hospital, Emily's response demonstrated that SDB had been an important feature of hospital admission, and with an awareness of the futility of professionals' attempts to keep her safe, stating

"I probably, yeah, got closer to s – killing myself in hospital than I did outside". Emily was aware that her SDB-use in hospital had multiple functions: "boredom, partly [laughing], but partly, [laughs] 'I'm gonna beat you'". She also emphasised the role of loss of agency, explaining that at the time she was thinking "I'm going to find a way, despite you taking away this, that and the other, I will find another way to do it".

"A couple of boxes of tablets, some dressings, razorblades, and your shopping"

Considering the all-consuming experience of Emily's engagement in SDB during her mid-twenties, it is conceivable her daily routines and patterns of occupational engagement are representative of a person whose primary occupation was engaging in SDB. Emily recalled a period of her life when her use of SDB had escalated but she was able to continue working full-time. Emily explained that each day it would be "just a case of getting home, run [laughs], perhaps eat [laughs], and then drink lots of alcohol". The use of "just a case" demonstrated the routine and regular nature of SDB, while laughter – when describing exercise and food-related occupations – was common throughout the interview.

Emily also clarified that certain types of SDB occurred at specific times of day; for example, alcohol-use was at night, overdosing of medication was at the weekend (in order not to negatively affect her work), whereas cutting was something that could happen during the day. This pattern suggests that her SDB-use was adapted in such a way that supported her ability to participate in her valued occupation of work. However, Emily was conscious that her SDB-use was unsustainable, stating "it's not possible for it to last", and found that the incongruence between how she was appearing and functioning at work, and her engagement in SDB as soon as she left work, could not be maintained.

Emily demonstrated awareness of the contrasts in her life now, posing the question: "I just didn't have anything in my life, did I?" In addition to this, she was describing SDB as a normalised behaviour, and yet with hindsight was somewhat incredulous at this occurrence. Emily explained how ensuring she had the supplies for SDB became normal – regular occupations in their own right; this was evident when she described how her grocery shopping had altered to "just put a, you know, a couple of boxes of tablets in there, some dressings, razorblades, and, then, your shopping! [laughs]". She had insight into the priority of these items over her usual groceries, appearing amused by how normal that behaviour seemed at the time.

"It stopped things in my head"

The reasons for use of SDB that Emily described were varied, with the most discussed being to manage stress; this was particularly related to having a demanding job with high levels of responsibility and difficult events happening within her family. SDB had a range of functions for Emily. For instance, her use of SDB in secret not only supported performance in valued occupations, but also served to release difficult emotions and manage stress: "it was my, kind of, release, being all normal-ish on the outside and then being able to manage that extra stress".

Additionally, Emily spoke about SDB being used to pass time. While she made reference to the partial function of SDB being to manage boredom in hospital, it had a differing mechanism for passing time at home, more akin to a means of escaping high levels of distress. Emily explained she "just wanted to drink to pass the time, and get rid of s – thoughts" and "it stopped things in my head", highlighting simultaneous functions of SDB to pass time, while providing escape from difficult thoughts.

Discussion: Emily's meaning, value, and purpose of participation in self-defeating behaviour

The term "self-defeating behaviour" was used throughout the interview due to it being a term more common in clinical settings. However, there was evidence that Emily's use and description of varied self-defeating behaviours would suggest these should be explored and understood as occupations. Emily spoke of her SDB-use as having a goal of destruction, shaping her identity as someone who "just self-harms", and providing a range of activities that she chose to participate in throughout the day. This finding mirrors long-recognised understandings of occupation as all of the activities that a person participates in throughout the day (Clark et al., 1991), with defining features of being "self-initiated, self-organised activity which is goal directed … and contextualised in a specific environment over a span of time" (Yerxa, 2000, p. 91).

Emily described self-defeating occupations as having "purpose". The long-established components of therapeutic occupation are activities that have both meaning and purpose (Trombly, 1995), but Emily's perspective provides insight that when occupations are not health-enhancing it may be easier to understand their purpose, whereas meaning may still have associations with the "positive".

While full understanding of the value of self-defeating occupations was not apparent to Emily, consideration of Emily's subjective experience and the value of self-defeating occupations, along with its "fit" with traditional concepts of occupation and health, provided insight into why it was so all-encompassing. For Emily, it supported goals of destruction and punishment, while providing her with a range of activities she was motivated to engage with. Yerxa (1998, p. 417) proposed that health could be "perceived as possession of a repertoire of skills enabling people to achieve their valued goals in their own environments". For Emily, while her goal was not a health-enhancing one, it was certainly a valued goal. The effect of self-defeating occupations on her health is less clear – she was aware of the consequences of alcohol abuse or overdose on her physical health, but it is not as easy to determine whether self-defeating occupations improved or worsened her mental well-being. I propose that an occupation with clear functions, including temporary reduction of distress, while not health-promoting, could be understood as a valued method of reducing emotional harm.

Limitations

The research presented was always intended to be exploratory in nature and a basis for larger studies which may clarify, develop, and expand our understanding of self-defeating occupations. The full study comprises greater analysis using occupational science constructs which has not been presented here. A single case study cannot represent the meaning and value of the many and varied occupations that are considered self-defeating for *all* people who live with BPD or Complex PTSD. However, it lays down the challenge that there is a wealth of understanding to be gained about the experience of living a life engaged in occupations often overlooked because of their self-destructive and non-health-promoting outcomes. Twinley (2016) found that maladaptive reactions to surviving sexual victimisation were explored and understood from the conceptual perspective of the "dark side of occupation", as they are "not extrinsically healthy, or restorative, but it could be that they are performed as survival occupations" (p. 257). I suggest there is an argument that the concept of survival occupations has resonance to those living with BPD or Complex PTSD.

Implications

Larger-scale research will further elucidate the experiences of people who engage in self-defeating occupations. The next challenges will be to determine how this knowledge can influence occupational therapy interventions, how people can be enabled to talk about self-defeating occupations, and, ultimately, enabling people to develop lives filled with more health-sustaining (and even health-promoting) occupations. As Twinley, Jacobs, and Clarke highlight in Chapter 20: "We need to consider the environments we work in and the extent to which they are conducive to having these (potentially) less comfortable or, even, more open discussions."

My personal experience was that exploring the complexity of the self-defeating occupations I used allowed me to understand why they were so powerful, and also why it initially appeared so difficult to replace, or change them, for self-sustaining occupations. The latter can be challenging, both for the person using the self-defeating occupations, and the occupational therapist, as the reality is that any "replacement" occupations are, initially at least, unlikely to have the same level of meaning and value. Moving away from reliance on self-defeating occupations is often a slow and gradual process, with setbacks, and sometimes the awareness of the magnitude of change required can be overwhelming. That said, the continued relative omission of an occupational perspective of self-defeating occupations upholds an inauthentic understanding of the person and their situation; I suggest this limits opportunities for meaningful and sustainable change.

Conclusion

People living with BPD are likely to have a long and rich occupational history involving a variety of occupations that could be understood as "self-defeating". In order to understand the person, and their occupational lives, attention needs to be paid to the dark side of occupation: occupations such as those I have discussed in the chapter. The process of change is far from straightforward and it is suggested that more research needs to be conducted about both the experience of engagement in the occupations and the means by which people can be supported to transition to occupations which sustain or, even, develop, rather than defeat, a person's health and well-being.

References

Baumeister, R., & Scher, S. (1988). Self-defeating behavior patterns among normal individuals: Review and analysis of common self-destructive tendencies. *Psychological Bulletin*, 104(1), 3–22. doi:10.1037/0033-2909.104.1.3.

Baxter, P., & Jack, S. (2008). Qualitative case study methodology: Study design and implementation for novice researchers. *The Qualitative Report*, 13(4), pp. 544–559. Retrieved from https://nsuworks.nova.edu/tqr/vol13/iss4/2

Clark, F., Parham, D., Carlson, M., Frank, G., Jackson, J., Pierce, D., ... Zemke, R. (1991). Occupational science: Academic innovation in the service of occupational therapy's future. *The American Journal of Occupational Therapy*, 45(4), 300–310. https://doi.org/10.5014/ajot.45.4.300.

Dallmayr, F. (2009). Hermeneutics and inter-cultural dialog: Linking theory and practice. *Ethics & Global Politics*, 2, 23–39. https://doi.org/10.3402/egp.v2i1.1937.

Denscombe, M. (2010). *The good research guide: For small-scale social research projects* (4th ed.). Maidenhead: McGraw-Hill/Open University Press.

DePoy, E., & Gitlin, L. (2011). *Introduction to research: Understanding and applying multiple strategies* (4th ed.). St. Louis, MO: Elsevier.

Gallop, R. (1992). Self-destructive and impulsive behavior in the patient with a borderline personality disorder: Rethinking hospital treatment and management. *Archives of Psychiatric Nursing*, 6(3), 178–182. http://dx.doi.org/10.1016/0883-9417(92)90029-I.

Palmer, R.E. (1969). *Hermeneutics: Interpretation theory in Schleiermacher, Dilthey, Heidegger, Gadamer*. Evanston, IL: Northwestern University Press.

Polit, D., & Beck, C. (2012). *Nursing research: Generating and assessing evidence for nursing practice* (9th ed.). Philadelphia: Wolters Kluwer Health/Lippincott Williams & Wilkins.

Smith, J. (2004). Reflecting on the development of interpretative phenomenological analysis and its contribution to qualitative research in psychology. *Qualitative Research in Psychology*, 1(1), 39–54. doi:10.1191/1478088704qp004oa.

Smith, J., Flowers, P., & Larkin, M. (2010). *Interpretative Phenomenological Analysis: Theory, method and research*. London: Sage.

Trombly, C. (1995). 1995 Eleanor Clarke Slagle Lecture – Occupation: Purposefulness and meaningfulness as therapeutic mechanisms. *American Journal of Occupational Therapy*, 49(10), 960–972. doi:10.5014/ajot.49.10.960.

Twinley, R. (2016). The perceived impacts of woman-to-woman rape and sexual assault, and the subsequent experience of disclosure, reaction, and support on victim/survivors' subjective experience of occupation (Doctoral dissertation, University of Plymouth, UK). Retrieved from https://pearl.plymouth.ac.uk/handle/10026.1/6551.

Twinley, R., & Addidle, G. (2012). Considering violence: The dark side of occupation. *British Journal of Occupational Therapy*, 75(4), 202–204. https://doi.org/10.4276/030802212X13336366278257.

Wasmuth, S., Crabtree, J.L., & Scott, P.J. (2014). Exploring addiction-as-occupation. *British Journal of Occupational Therapy*, 77(12), 605–613. doi:10.4276/030802214X14176260335264.

Yerxa, E. (1998). Health and the human spirit for occupation. *American Journal of Occupational Therapy*, 52(6), 412–418. https://doi.org/10.5014/ajot.52.6.412.

Yerxa, E. (2000). Occupational science: A renaissance of service to humankind through knowledge. *Occupational Therapy International*, 7(2), 87–98. doi:10.1002/oti.109.

9 Exploring the impact of childhood sexual abuse trauma in the context of the occupation of work

S. Caroline Taylor

Background

Childhood sexual abuse (CSA) and its array of impacts are well established in scholarly literature as well as through the voices of victim/survivors themselves (Cashmore & Shackle, 2013; Taylor, Pugh, Goodwach, & Coles, 2012). The important and hard-earned social and political conscious-ness raising about CSA that has occurred over the last four decades has been largely driven by feminist activism and scholarship. These actions have led to significant sociopolitical, legal, and criminal justice reforms, and have enabled survivor-led activism to influence political action. For instance, in Australia, Ireland, the USA, and the UK, various governments have established inquiries and Royal Commissions to examine the sexual abuse of children in religious and government institutions – deliberately avoiding the institution of the family, where the majority of child sexual abuse occurs. The politics of child sexual abuse remain such that the vast majority of victim/survivors – specifically those children sexually abused within the family unit – remain politically and socially silenced and/or mar-ginalised. The further implications of this being that these children, who often remain in vulnerable circumstances, need substantial efforts and support to achieve social and occupational justice (Hocking, 2017).

Trauma and occupation

Trauma and its immediate and residual impacts have been linked to socio-economic disadvantages across the lifespan for victim/survivors, and this includes educational attainment. With literature well establishing the impacts upon health for victim/survivors, there is limited research focused on socio-economic and occupational (work) disadvantages created as a consequence of CSA (Barrett, Kamiya, & O'Sullivan, 2014; Goodman, Joyce, & Smith, 2011; Robst & VanGilder, 2011). Available studies (such as those previously cited) highlight CSA trauma and its impact on education outcomes, obstacles to employment, reduced workforce participation, lower income levels, and difficulties in work performance as a consequence of CSA-related mental health issues. These studies have value for illuminating another layer of trauma consequence connected to employment opportunity and access, as well as income and financial well-being. However there remains a deeper complexity to this burgeoning file and that is the relationship between the survivor and their workplace as a site for re-traumatisation and re-victimisation.

Consistent with her concept of the dark side of occupation, Twinley's (2016) doctoral research was an endeavour to explore an unspoken area of sexual victimisation; in this work she offers a rich insight into the experiences for women survivors of female sexual offending and the negative emotional impacts on their occupations. For people with enduring mental health issues including a diagnosis of PTSD, work as a meaningful and productive occupation (and other productive occupations) enables the development of occupational identity, routine, and structure, which are helpful in building confidence and feelings of safety, as well as a sense of belonging (Whalley Hammell, 2017). As such, work (as occupation) provides more than economic benefit (Twinley, 2016). Notwithstanding these benefits, Twinley's interviews with adult women survivors revealed work disruption due to ongoing trauma and its attendant impact on work performance, satisfaction, and the hiatus between having a job and being unable to work due to trauma. Participants in her research detailed the intrusion of triggers in their work-related occupations, as well as negative coping strategies such as substance abuse which impacted job performance and ability to sustain employment (Twinley, 2017).

Aside from Twinley's contribution, the complex intersection of sexual violence, particularly CSA, and work occupations is an under-researched area in urgent need of attention to uncover what many survivors and some professionals who work with survivors know – and that is the residual trauma and associated triggers that negatively affect the spectrum of work and other "productive" occupations. The concept of "social death" has been applied in my early work on CSA (Taylor, 2004) and built on substantially through funded and ongoing research that is the subject of a forthcoming book. My research involved in-depth interviews with 78 female and male CSA victim/survivors with a focus on post-abuse experiences of rebuilding, recovery, trauma impact, non-finite grief, and post-traumatic growth. One area of my data that has specific relevance to this chapter is the significant impact on work experienced by victim/survivors in my study. My forthcoming book provides occupational therapists, scientists, and others with a valuable opportunity to explore the potential for workplaces be a trigger for victim/survivors, making them fraught places of occupation.

I also found that workplaces can be a place where victims are targeted, especially those who present with vulnerabilities associated with a history of CSA, or indeed when others have knowledge of the victim/survivor's history as a victim.[1] The majority of victim/survivors do not disclose the abuse, or do so many years later, and many report negative reactions to their disclosures. Either way, these silences and negative responses exacerbate victim trauma and should remind everyone of the daily courage shown by victim/survivors to face each and every day of their lives; this includes seeking work and care for themselves and others in a world where their own suffering is often unseen or misunderstood or ignored.

Uncovering the potential for re-traumatisation at work

Many participants in my study spoke of making vocational/occupational choices they believed would either aid them in their recovery or provide an environment to shield them from their traumatic memories.

"Ryan"

In Ryan's[2] case he believed that his aggressive anger outbursts, that developed following his sexual abuse by a teacher in primary school, would find supportive expression in the army where he perceived hyper-masculinity and visible strength and toughness were accepted. He thought his occupational choice with its imposed routine, structure, and hyper-masculinity would restore his fragile sense of self and his belief that presenting to the world as "a tough man" would protect him from his own wounds of CSA. However, his trauma-related issues began to clash with his work and other occupations in the army. Ryan identified his uncontrolled anger outbursts as a major issue, along with his inability to accept direction from supervisors as they reminded him of the authority figure of his childhood abuser. He was dishonourably discharged and told me it took him more than 10 years to overcome this period of his life, during which time he experienced long periods of unemployment with short-term work.

"Sarah"

Another participant, Sarah, developed in childhood what she later understood were "panic attacks", at night-time. The debilitating nature of these attacks impacted with Sarah's vocational dream of being a nurse at a time when nurses trained on-site in a hospital setting. She had been a high performing student in her studies and exams and recalled how she utilised various coping mechanisms to suppress her panic attacks. However, her second clinical ward placement required her to do some rostered night shifts. Sarah found she could not control her panic attacks and her behaviour came to the attention of staff. Unable to properly explain what she was experiencing and feeling unable to disclose her history of CSA because of stigma-threat (see Gibson & Leitenberg, 2001; Miller, Canales, Amacker, Backstrom, & Gidycz, 2011), Sarah reports that she began to lose confidence in her work and in her study. Moreover, she felt misjudged, which exacerbated her anxiety. Before the end of her first year of nursing, Sarah resigned from her paid nurse training.

For many participants in my study, the workplace was fraught with triggers causing deleterious emotional impacts, leading some to leave their job or vocational career, or to develop, in many cases, maladaptive coping mechanisms, to try and cope with being in the workplace. I uncovered stories of victim/survivors trialling self-developed remedies to try and cope with their work or hold on to their employment or vocational training/study. Workplace performance issues, job dissatisfaction or untenable tensions with management or other colleagues were a frequent reality that led to disrupted work histories, unemployment, loss of confidence and self-esteem, exacerbated trauma, and financial problems. What was clear from these experiences was the lack of understanding and support in the workplace. Occupation is understood as a means to express ourselves and to achieve a sense of belonging and connectedness (Whalley Hammell, 2014), meaning the findings in my study highlight the need for the relative scholarly silence of this phenomenon to be illuminated and explored in further ventures.

Crisis-driven disclosure

The brave decision by some victim/survivors to disclose to their workplace supervisor in the hope of securing understanding and support did not prove helpful.

"Julia"

Julia recalls how workplace triggers that affected her trauma memories led to severe anxiety. She had worked very hard to obtain an undergraduate degree in her chosen vocational field and in her first job found herself triggered by a project she was working on with colleagues. Unable to cope, Julia made what I have termed a "crisis driven disclosure" (Muldoon, Taylor, & Norma, 2016; Taylor, Muldoon, Norma, & Bradley, 2012; Taylor & Norma, 2013) to her supervisor in the hope of securing support for her noticed workplace distress. Instead, her supervisor rebuked her for "oversharing" personal information that he believed was not relevant to the workplace, and so felt it best to remove her from the assigned project. The negative reaction to Julia's disclosure and her removal from her project role led to what Julia described as a "mental and emotional downward spiralling". Negative reactions to victim/survivor disclosures and their link to compounding trauma, PTSD symptoms, and delayed recovery is well established in scholarly research (Littleton, 2010; Orchowski, Untied, & Gidycz, 2013; Ullman, 2007). In Julia's case it also compromised her trust and confidence in her supervisor, who she feared might share her disclosure with others. This made Julia feel unsafe and unsupported in her workplace and she doubted her own skills and ability to contribute to her chosen profession; her sense of belonging was undeniably compromised.

Julia's work in her chosen vocation, for which she had worked hard to make it a reality, became a daily struggle as the distress increasingly impacted her work performance and collegial relationships, with absenteeism and self-exclusion from work colleagues as her coping strategies for survival. Over the next two months Julia's supervisor restricted her work role and, in a private conversation, indicated to Julia that he felt her "lack of boundaries" in raising her childhood history, coupled with what was described as her "emotional state" at work, required him to limit her work projects as a form of workplace safety for others. For Julia, these comments and actions defeated her fragile grasp in her work employment. Soon after, Julia resigned and never again sought to work in her profession. I witnessed how recalling the work aspect of her occupational life was clearly an area of ongoing distress and grief for Julia. She described feelings of wasted years at university; being robbed of a future in a profession that would have enabled her to travel and apply her vocational passion. Ongoing feelings of humiliation, shame, worthlessness, and failure remained trauma markers in her life.

"Thomas"

Thomas experienced CSA that most often occurred in an underground cellar. The trauma negatively impacted his educational attainment and he experienced anxiety attacks. Thomas secured work at a large retail store. Due to a sudden staff shortage Thomas was asked to assist working in the cellar storeroom which was located below ground and was quite a dark and quiet place. The impact of this environment upon his well-being was sudden; this work location triggered serious flashbacks for Thomas, and he endured anxiety attacks leading to work performance issues and work absenteeism. In fear of losing his job, Thomas approached his supervisor requesting that he work back on the main retail floor and not in the storeroom. His request was denied. Thomas disclosed in confidence to the manager of retail staff that he had a history of CSA and could not work in the cellar area. Without his permission, his manager advised the store supervisor of Thomas' disclosure and he became aware that this information had become known to other staff. Whilst Thomas was no longer required to work in the cellar, this violation of his confidential disclosure and accompanying comments by staff led to further anxiety attacks about his workplace in general, and he soon left this employment.

"Melinda"

Melinda worked in the public sector and experienced sexual and non-sexual harassment by two male employees and a female employee, each of whom were more senior in their roles. Fearful of reporting the sexual harassment, and experiencing triggers to her CSA, Melinda sought employee-assisted counselling, but found it unhelpful. She employed coping mechanisms, such as seeking transfer to another department and utilising sick leave. Her symptoms of distress escalated leaving her feeling isolated as the harassment continued, and her inability to hide her anxiety and fear at work led to comments that she was not mentally stable. This commentary added to her distress and anxiety and Melinda went on long-term sick leave. Feeling trapped and unable to return to work, Melinda made a claim of workplace bullying. As with Sarah, she felt unable to disclose her CSA and the sexual harassment at the hands of male employees and so her claim revolved around the bullying and harassment. Her claim was rejected. Melinda resigned and reported that the impact on her mental health was such that she remained out of the workforce for the next five years.

Bullying and harassment of CSA victim/ survivors at work

Workplace bullying, harassment, and discrimination is a significant issue in modern workplaces across the globe, with recognised health consequences for those exposed to such conduct (Chan-Mok, Caponecchia, & Winder, 2014; Okechukwu, Souza, Davis, & de Castro, 2014). Research on workplace bullying and mobbing suggests certain character traits[3] such as lower self-esteem, anxiety, and poorly developed social and coping skills (Nielsen & Einarsen, 2018) heightened chances of being targeted in the workplace (Glasø, Matthiesen, Nielson, & Einarsen, 2007; Shallcross, Sheehan, & Ramsay, 2008).

Healthcare professionals have begun to pay more attention to people who present with physiological and mental health issues as a consequence of workplace bullying and harassment and who have a history of CSA.[4] Those with an expertise in CSA are recognising a strong link with workplace harassment and bullying as a significant trigger, causing aspects of the emotional trauma from childhood to resurface and compound the workplace trauma. In some cases, victims of workplace bullying and harassment (sexual and non-sexual) become conscious of the trigger relationship, whilst others may not. In either scenario, there is a likelihood for these people to develop serious and enduring physical and health issues that, to the untrained eye, may seem disproportionate to the original workplace incident/s. This doubling of the original childhood trauma in the workplace can complicate diagnosis because of the complex health sequalae, in addition to treatment (or intervention), and an appreciation of the seriousness of the present-ing trauma symptomology. Growing awareness amongst practising healthcare professionals has led them to actively explore a history of CSA with a person presenting with serious trauma-related health prob-lems stemming from workplace bullying and harassment. As Twinley asserted, there is

> [a] need for an occupational perspective of diversity, injustice, alien-ation, and other such concerns affecting marginalised, minority, and vulnerable groups. Addressing the needs of such groups – including those who experience trauma-related symptoms and posttraumatic stress disorder (PTSD) – has the potential to improve the effectiveness of services provided by rehabilitation professionals.
>
> (2017, p. 509)

Workplace triggers for victim/survivors of CSA may be unintentional in that they are part of the occupational tasks performed in the work. Triggers caused by workplace bullying and harassment can and do have catastrophic impacts for victim/survivors with a history of CSA and this remains a relat-ively hidden area of research that requires attention.

Human rights and justice

Given the global statistics on childhood sexual abuse, the reality is that every workplace more than likely has employees living their daily, occupa-tional lives with residual trauma. Dignity in the workplace is an essential human right for everyone. Its absence impacts individual and collective well-being and productivity. The stories of victim/survivors of CSA making choices to avoid trauma triggers at work, or tenuously holding on to employment or study despite unintended triggers, or those caused by work-place bullying and harassment, ought to remind everyone of the resolute courage they display in their journeys to survive, thrive, and engage in meaningful occupation and belonging. Trauma associated with a history of CSA and other forms of sexual victimisation is an invisible victim/survivor burden and is a barrier to the "doing" occupations of paid employment and educational pursuits (Whalley Hammell, 2009). As workplaces around the world develop and enact inclusion and anti-discrimination policies for sexual orientation, race, gender, disability, and religion, there is a gaping hole with regard to those who experience enduring health sequalae from CSA; people who live with this impact experience both discrimination and a negation of their "doing" occupations of work or of study endeavours. It remains an invisible, or dark side, of occupation (as understood and explored by occupational therapists and scientists), occupational health, and of human rights at work.

Conclusion

The workplace should be an environment that positively supports either recovery or coping by providing a safe workplace and one that is trauma-informed. It is clear that victim/survivors of CSA experience health and socio-economic barriers to meaningful employment and the pursual of educational and vocational goals and dreams. Moreover, residual trauma that impacts their health and well-being intersects with the occupation of work, in addition to other aspects of daily occupation. Workplace bullying and harassment is a serious issue for every business, organisation, and person in the workforce. Of great concern, the capacity for workplace bullying and harassment to trigger and generate relapse of an earlier trauma, that is compounded by workplace trauma, remains an area in need of urgent attention by (amongst others) researchers, clinicians, lawyers, occupational therapists, and policy makers.

Notes

1 With regard to the latter point, there is not the scope in this chapter to discuss the data in my research where participants described intentional targeting of themselves based on knowledge of their history of CSA. This was especially so for participants who were successful in their career or who were deemed different from the broader organisational culture. It was also raised negatively to question participants who sought to report sexual harassment or other forms of discrimination and harassment.

2 Note that pseudonyms are used for each participant. The research drawn upon in this chapter is the subject of a forthcoming book to be published by Spinifex Press.

3 Traits which have been identified as vulnerabilities in employment status for those with a history of CSA.

4 I am indebted to Dr Sandra Hacker, AO, a highly respected psychiatrist based in Melbourne, Australia, for her invaluable insights that support my commentary regarding clinical awareness of CSA and its links with workplace trauma.

References

Barrett, A., Kamiya, Y., & O'Sullivan, V. (2014). The long-term impact of childhood sexual abuse on incomes and labour force status. Papers RB2014/3/1, Economic and Social Research Institute (ESRI). Retrieved from https://ideas.repec.org/p/esr/wpaper/rb2014-3-1.html.

Cashmore, J., & Shackle, R. (2013). The long-term effects of child sexual abuse. CFCA Paper No. 11. Melbourne, Australia: Australian Institute of Family Studies. Retrieved from https://aifs.gov.au/cfca/publications/long-term-effects-child-sexual-abuse.

Chan-Mok, J.O., Caponecchia, C., & Winder, C. (2014). The concept of workplace bullying: Implications from Australian workplace health and safety law. *Psychiatry, Psychology and the Law, 21*(3), pp. 442–456. https://doi.org/10.1080/13218719.2013.829399.

Gibson, L.E., & Leitenberg, H. (2001). The impact of child sexual abuse and stigma on methods of coping with sexual assault among undergraduate women. *Child Abuse and Neglect*, 25, pp. 1343–1361. doi:10.1016/s0145-2134(01)00279-4.

Glasø, L., Matthiesen, S.B., Nielson, M.B., & Einarsen, S. (2007). Do targets of workplace bullying portray a general victim personality profile? *Scandinavian Journal of Psychology*, 48(4), pp. 313–319. https://doi.org/10.1111/j.1467-9450.2007.00554.x.

Goodman, A., Joyce, R., & Smith, J.P. (2011). The long shadow cast by childhood physical and mental problems on adult life. *Proceedings of the National Academy of Sciences of the United States of America*, 108(15), pp. 6032–6037. doi:10.1073/pnas.1016970108.

Hocking, C. (2017). Occupational justice as social justice: The moral claim for inclusion. *Journal of Occupational Science*, 24(1), pp. 29–42. doi:10.1080/14427591.2017.1294016.

Littleton, H.L. (2010). The impact of social support and negative disclosure reactions on sexual assault victims: A cross-sectional and longitudinal investigation. *Journal of Trauma & Dissociation*, 11(2), pp. 210–227. doi:10.1080/152997309 03502946.

Miller, A.K., Canales, E.J., Amacker, A.M., Backstrom, T.L., & Gidycz, C.A. (2011). Stigma-threat motivated nondisclosure of sexual assault and sexual revictimization: A prospective analysis. *Psychology of Women Quarterly*, 35(1), pp. 119–128. https://doi.org/10.1177/0361684310384104.

Muldoon, S.D., Taylor, S.C., & Norma, C. (2016). The survivor master narrative in sexual assault. *Violence Against Women: An International, Interdisciplinary Journal*, 22(5), pp. 565–587. https://doi.org/10.1177/1077801215608701.

Nielsen, M.B., & Einarsen, S.V. (2018). What we know, what we do not know, and what we should and could have known about workplace bullying: An overview of the literature and agenda for future research. *Aggression and Violent Behavior*, 42, pp. 71–83. https://doi.org/10.1016/j.avb.2018.06.007.

Okechukwu, C.A., Souza, K., Davis, K.D., & de Castro, A.B. (2014). Discrimination, harassment, abuse and bullying in the workplace: Contribution of workplace injustice to occupational health disparities. *American Journal of Industrial Medicine*, 57(5), pp. 573–568. doi:10.1002/ajim.22221.

Orchowski, L.M., Untied, A.S., & Gidycz, C.A. (2013). Social reactions to disclosure of sexual victimization and adjustment among survivors of sexual assault. *Journal of Interpersonal Violence*, 28(10), pp. 2005–2023. doi:10.1177/0886260512471085.

Robst, J., & VanGilder, J. (2011). The role of childhood sexual victimization in the occupational choice of adults. *Applied Economics*, 43(3), pp. 341–354. doi:10.1080/00036840802584893.

Shallcross, L., Sheehan, M., & Ramsay, S. (2008). Workplace mobbing: Experiences in the public sector. *Workplace Mobbing: Experiences in the Public Sector*, 13(2), pp. 56–70. Retrieved from https://core.ac.uk/download/pdf/10905480.pdf.

Taylor, S.C. (2004). *Court licensed abuse*. New York: Peter Lang.

Taylor, S.C., Muldoon, S.D., Norma, C., & Bradley, D. (2012). Policing just outcomes: Improving the police response to adults reporting sexual assault. Retrieved from https://trove.nla.gov.au/work/181577925.

Taylor, S.C., & Norma, C. (2013). The ties that bind: Family barriers for adult women seeking to report childhood sexual assault in Australia. *Women's Studies International Forum*, 37, pp. 114–124. https://doi.org/10.1016/j.wsif.2012.11.004.

Taylor, S.C., Pugh, J., Goodwach, R., & Coles, J. (2012). Sexual trauma in women – the importance of identifying a history of sexual violence. *Australian Family Physician*, 41(7), pp. 538–541.

Twinley, R. (2016). The perceived impacts of woman-to-woman rape and sexual assault, and the subsequent experience of disclosure, reaction, and support on victim/survivors' subjective experience of occupation (Doctoral dissertation, University of Plymouth, UK). Retrieved from https://pearl.plymouth.ac.uk/handle/10026.1/6551.

Twinley, R. (2017). Woman-to-woman rape and sexual assault, and its impact upon the occupation of work: Victim/survivors' life roles of worker or student as disruptive and preservative. *Work*, 56(4), pp. 505–517. doi:10.3233/WOR-172529.

Ullman, S.E. (2007). Relationship to perpetrator, disclosure, social reactions, and PTSD symptoms in child sexual abuse survivors. *Journal of Child Sexual Abuse*, 16(1), pp. 16–36. https://doi.org/10.1300/J070v16n01_02.

Whalley Hammell, K. (2009). Self-care, productivity, and leisure, or dimensions of occupational experience? Rethinking occupational "categories". *Canadian Journal of Occupational Therapy*, 76(2), pp. 107–114. https://doi.org/10.1177/000841740907600208.

Whalley Hammell, K. (2014). Belonging, occupation, and human well-being: An exploration. *Canadian Journal of Occupational Therapy*, 81(1), pp. 39–50. doi:10.1177/0008417413520489.

Whalley Hammell, K. (2017). Opportunities for well-being: The right to occupational engagement. *Canadian Journal of Occupational Therapy*, 84(4–5), pp. 209–222. doi:10.1177/0008417417734831.

Part III

Occupational therapy practice

10 Challenges for occupational therapists working with clients who choose illicit, immoral or health-compromising occupations

Craig Greber

Professional reasoning in occupational therapy

Through a process of information gathering, synthesis and intervention, occupational therapists are able to manage complicated issues to enhance participation in occupation for their clients (American Occupational Therapy Association, 2014). Studies of professional reasoning in occupational therapy have enabled the profession to systematically approach the challenge of working with diverse individuals and populations from an occupation-focused perspective. Using an expansive reasoning process enables clinicians to engage effectively in decision-making, however the complex nature of problem-solving in occupational therapy prevents the adoption of formulaic thinking (Robertson & Griffiths, 2012). The myriad factors a therapist skilfully balances when working with a client often lead to novel ways of thinking that are best served by considering the situation in non-linear ways. As Chapparo and Ranka (2000) asserted, clinical reasoning in occupational therapy is characterised by the use of multiple reasoning strategies that consider the internal and external influences during client management. Boyt Schell and Benfield (2018) described these modes as "aspects of professional reasoning". Those authors identified five such aspects: scientific, narrative, pragmatic, ethical, and interactive reasoning. Each of these engages enquiry in different ways and contributes different perspectives to the therapist's thinking. Given the complexity of discussion regarding the place of illicit, immoral, and health-compromising occupations in the practice of occupational therapy, it is prudent to use this multimodal description of professional reasoning to consider the issue.

Understanding health and wellbeing – an application
of scientific reasoning

Scientific reasoning uses a systematic and logical approach to help therapists make decisions by using scientific method to understand evidence, recognise patterns, and generate and test hypotheses (Tomlin, 2018). A scientific perspective seeks to understand causal relationships and predict outcomes. It is largely impersonal and disregards a person's experiences, goals, and values (Tomlin, 2018). The application of scientific reasoning focuses the current discussion on two main issues: definitions of health and the relationship between health and occupation.

The International Classification of Functioning, Disability and Health (World Health Organization, 2001) described health in terms of three parameters: body functions and structure, activity, and participation. While occupational therapists are driven to endorse this broad definition, they frequently find their scope of practice constrained by more reductionist perspectives that focus exclusively on body structure and function in describing the health or otherwise of individuals. The challenge of narrower definitions of health is that they make it difficult to contemplate occasions when subjective experience of participation in activities brings about meaning, purpose and life satisfaction, but is concomitantly damaging or potentially damaging to body structure and function. Further, such definitions prove troublesome when an occupation is health-promoting in certain contexts, frequencies, and durations but unhealthy in others, or when the occupation supports some elements of health yet compromises others.

To some extent, the term "wellbeing" has been used to refocus discussion away from narrow definitions of health. However, like meaning and purpose, wellbeing is an individually derived construct, and so establishing a universal definition has proven difficult (Dodge, Daly, Huyton, & Sanders, 2012). The irony of narrower stances on health and wellbeing is that many behaviours that appear to be health-promoting or health-sustaining can become health-compromising in particular contexts. Those same things that enhance health – exercise, eating, exposure to sunlight and so on – can also erode health if not moderated in some way. As fundamental an occupation as eating can have health-compromising characteristics when particular foods form a disproportionate component of the diet, or when caloric intake is excessive. Some apparently health-sustaining occupations, such as hand washing, can even prove to become the subject of obsessive-compulsive behaviours when a person's mental health is challenged.

Accordingly, it is often difficult to confidently position occupations along a healthy–unhealthy continuum. What might be good for psychological health might compromise physiological health, or create risks to the personal safety of the person or their community. When considered holistically, there can be demonstrable benefits from smoking, drinking alcohol or consumption of illicit drugs in sustaining psychological, social, emotional and even physical health. When used in a balanced and respons-ible manner, a person might experience a sense of wellbeing that otherwise escapes them. For that reason, it has often proved difficult for occupational therapists to ascertain the extent to which an occupation is health-promoting, health-sustaining or health-compromising, let alone to decide how best to position themselves in working with clients to enable performance of those occupations.

Creek and Hughes (2008), through their systematic review of the liter-ature, reported that evidence of a relationship between occupation and health is considerable, but incomplete. While these authors concluded that occupation has been shown to directly influence health and wellbeing, the nature of that influence depends on characteristics of the occupation. The assumption that occupation necessarily enhances health was shown to be errant. It is therefore the skilled application of occupation that is the key to healthy outcomes; self-chosen occupations are less likely to result in health-oriented outcomes. And yet the drive to respond to client preferences is strong, creating philosophical and ethical tensions for clinicians when forced to choose between embracing client choice and redirecting clients towards occupations more commensurate with good health. Therapists endeavour not to impose their own values onto the choices their clients make, but are often uncomfortable about being complicit in promoting participation in occupations they do not believe are health-oriented. Man-aging such situations must therefore be based on understanding why clients might choose illicit, immoral or health-compromising occupations as a source of meaning and purpose.

Choosing occupational goals: understanding through narrative reasoning

A narrative is a story or perspective based on subjective, personalised ways of experiencing life (Hamilton, 2018). Narrative reasoning enables a therapist to understand a client's perspective by exploring their lived experiences, preferences, interests and lifestyle. By exploring a client's narrative, and the narratives of those close to them, a therapist is able to understand how par-ticular occupations impose meaning and purpose. The process of narrative reasoning also unearths client values, interests, relationships and experiences that are useful in planning the therapeutic process. This aspect of reasoning helps therapists understand how clients experience meaning and purpose through illegal, deviant or unhealthy occupations.

From previous work in the area, we can begin to glimpse the motivation of some clients to engage in behaviours that are illicit, immoral or detri-mental to health. Risk-taking has been characterised as a moderately stable trait across the lifespan, despite such behaviours peaking during adoles-cence (Josef et al., 2016). Several influential factors have been proposed, including affective, social and efficacious reinforcers (Aziz & Sumaira, 2018;

Van Hoorn, Fuligini, Erone, & Galvan, 2016), and emotional dysregulation (Weiss, Sullivan, & Tull, 2015). Unethical behaviour has long been thought to occur as the result of breakdown in the congruence between a person's moral judgement and their chosen behaviour, however Bersoff (1999) proposed that in some cases the desire for personal gain (either affective or material) corrupts a person's moral judgement, making the behaviour justifiable from an ethical standpoint. When combined with social reinforcement, illegal, immoral or unhealthy behaviours evolve as a new ethical norm through cognitive distortions (Szumski, Bartels, Beech, & Fisher, 2018). Similar influences have been proposed to contribute to the normalisation of violent behaviours (World Health Organization, 2002). Moral flexibility, it seems, can lead people to experience meaning and purpose through illegal, immoral or risky health behaviours.

Narrative reasoning enables a therapist to understand how a client experiences meaning and purpose through occupation. Despite acknowledging a narrative that describes why a client chooses particular occupations, the extent to which the therapist can support participation in those occupations is contentious and best understood through engaging other aspects of reasoning.

Considering what is possible: pragmatic reasoning

As much as therapists seek to develop interventions that serve client needs, they do so within the boundaries of everyday reality. Funding, equipment, time, protocols, and skills all conspire to limit the range of approaches a therapist might use. While other forms of reasoning generate potential solutions to a client's issues, those solutions must all prove viable within the context of the therapist's practice and the client's circumstances (Boyt Schell, 2018). Pragmatic reasoning not only determines what is possible, it also acknowledges the scope of practice and domain of concern. It forms an important way of understanding the practical constraints in managing the needs of a client with preferences for illicit, immoral or health-compromising occupations.

Employer organisations often constrain the way illicit, immoral or health-compromising client goals can be addressed. Service funding parameters dictate anticipated outcomes and when client goals do not match those, it becomes difficult for clinicians to reconcile discrepancies between the client's goals and the organisation's responsibilities. While a clinician might seek to embrace a client's choice to prioritise particular occupations, the extent to which they can do so is often imposed from elsewhere.

Doing what is right: ethical reasoning

When therapists consider how best to enable clients to perform target occupations, there are inevitable limits to what should reasonably be done in a given situation. The process of exploring what is reasonable and just has been labelled ethical reasoning (Slater, Doherty, & Erler, 2018). Ethical reasoning provides a means of objectively considering issues of morality, values, and legal implications associated with practice, including consideration of any dissonance between the therapist's own morality and that of his/ her client.

Ethical reasoning enables clinicians to consider not just what is evidence-based, what the client might want, or what might be possible in the context of service delivery, but also what *should* be done from an ethical standpoint. It is founded on basic ethical principles, primarily the responsibility to do good for the client and resisting doing harm. High quality services should be provided in ways that are in accordance with professional codes of ethics and relevant legislation, yet establish shared knowledge and treat in accordance with the client's wishes.

Legislation is often enacted within societies to articulate and uphold moral codes. For clinicians, the presence of legislation can simplify the ethical reasoning process. Mandatory reporting requirements, for example, can simplify decisions about how to manage occasions where clients reveal information about some forms of illegal activity. But these requirements are not universal and clinicians are frequently left to make independent judgements. There is reason to turn instead to the professional code of ethics for guidance. Such codes are based on ethical foundations and, while they provide an ethical starting point, they often fail to provide clear guidance on how best to proceed. For that reason, a more comprehensive process for engaging in ethical reasoning is required.

Taking an ethical stance when a client identifies occupations that are morally questionable would appear to be a straightforward response to the dilemma of working with clients who find meaning and purpose in immoral acts; however, morality itself is an inherently subjective construct. An individual's ethical standpoint is derived in part from cultural, religious, and organisational beliefs. One of the challenges of making ethical decisions is that the societal values that underpin them are constantly changing. In many cultures, more liberal stances evolve that challenge long-held values and morals. It is reasonable to expect, then, that therapists and their clients might not share the same ethical perspectives regarding participation in occupation. The therapist's and client's morality must feature equally in ethical decision-making (Chapparo & Ranka, 2000).

Dealing with extremes of behaviour is an easier ethical decision than managing the uncomfortable areas in between. While ethical reasoning might be relatively easy to apply when a client seeks to engage in an occupation with severe known and pervasive health risks or in breach of laws, it is more challenging to reach conclusions about those things that are only mildly unhealthy, morally questionable or are unhealthy only when moderation is exceeded. Ethical dilemmas also loom when an occupation might contribute positively to one element of health, yet impact negatively on another. There is simply no ethical prescription that can inform clinicians in dealing with such instances. Instead, ethical reasoning must be synthesised with other aspects of reasoning to determine an appropriate action.

Client-centred practice: collaboration through interactive reasoning

Turpin and Copley (2018) proposed interactive reasoning as a means of working with clients through the skilful application of the therapeutic relationship. Interactive reasoning involves working collaboratively with the client towards a shared vision of hope for the future. While engagement with clients can provide a means of gathering information to support other aspects of professional reasoning, it more importantly serves as an avenue for understanding the whole of the client's situation and a forum for collaborating on solutions.

While occupational therapists have long placed the client at the centre of decision-making, it is important to acknowledge that it would be irresponsible for clinicians to mindlessly accede to the demands of clients without at least drawing the client into conversations about their choices. Occupational therapists are able to reflect, acknowledge, educate, understand, and challenge the benefits, or otherwise, of occupations without compromising principles of client-centredness. Blindly accepting client directives without providing a professional perspective on them is unhelpful, irresponsible, and unethical.

When a client nominates or identifies an occupational goal, they do so from the perspective of personal experience, knowledge, interest, and exposure. Espoused occupational goals are restricted as well as facilitated by these factors, and they often represent limited consideration of alternative or equivalent occupations that could impose meaning and purpose in ways that meet the client's needs. When client-identified occupations do not match professional responsibilities to enable health and wellbeing through occupation, practitioners can discuss these occupations with the client to identify alternative ways of meeting these needs. It is not sufficient to become obedient to a client's espoused wishes without working with the client to understand the drive behind those occupations, and the meaning and purpose experienced through them, and where appropriate to propose alternative ways of meeting occupational need.

It is reasonable to expect that while a client brings their own desires, experiences, and preferences to an encounter, there are occasions when that perspective might change with the addition of knowledge and information. Through interactive reasoning, the clinician shares a perspective with the client and together the therapist and client make decisions regarding goals, timeframes, and approaches (Turpin & Copley, 2018). While the needs of the client remain at the centre of discussions, the clinician contributes to decisions within their scope of practice. Therapists and clients are partners in decision-making and the therapeutic relationship provides the space for this collaboration. In some instances the distinction between client-centred and client-driven perspectives might be hard to draw, but the clinician has a professional responsibility to ensure decisions are made on an informed basis.

Professional reasoning – a complex response to a complex problem

Professional reasoning in occupational therapy requires the therapist to forge investigations, gather information, understand perspectives, recognise limits, draw conclusions, and make decisions. For clients who prioritise illicit, immoral or health-compromising occupations, a thorough professional reasoning process enables therapists to make appropriate decisions based on information about prognosis, client values and experiences, service resources and expectations, ethical and moral principles, and the therapeutic relationship. At the same time, this reasoning must be undertaken within the therapist's own knowledge of the power of meaningful occupation, and the theories that inform that knowledge.

It is overly simplistic to present occupational therapy as a means of returning clients to premorbid occupations. While that might be a reasonable outcome to anticipate in many cases, there are many more where the occupations identified by the client necessitate modification, adaptation, and even substitution. Clients receive services when life events have transpired to limit their participation in occupation. While a return to premorbid occupations might be viewed as ideal, there are occasions where a client's occupational interests can help identify new roles that provide meaning and purpose in ways that do not involve participation in those premorbid occupations. Opportunities exist to explore occupational interests beyond the client's lived experience of occupation. For clients who identify illicit, immoral or health-compromising occupations as targets for intervention, substituting one occupation with another can ensure that meaning and purpose continue to be experienced, without potential legal, moral or health-compromising consequences.

At the commencement of therapy, a client's stated occupational goal might not be commensurate with health or legal and moral standards and yet it provides an opportunity to interact with the client to explore occupational need. Skilled engagement with a client who identifies an illegal or health-compromising occupational goal can promote re-evaluation of that goal and potential substitution with another occupation that carries less physical, psychological, legal, and moral risk. Engaging in this way respects the motivation clients might have to engage in unhealthy, immoral or illegal occupations, but provides opportunities for self-exploration, discovery, and change.

Facilitating positive outcomes – an occupational therapy response

Occupational scientists seek to understand how people impose meaning and purpose through occupation, including occupations that are illegal, immoral or health-compromising. For occupational therapists, however, the concept of occupation is more exclusive, based on those things that might contribute positively to both the individual and the society in which they function. Occupational therapists seek to use occupation as a therapeutic tool that contributes broadly to the wellbeing of an individual, while at the same time conforming to the requirements of employer organisations, the professional code of ethics, and moral and legal expectations of the community. Occupational therapists are constrained in the way they construe unhealthy, immoral or illegal occupations, as well as the way they use those occupations to attain other gains for clients.

Clinicians negotiate this troublesome space by combining a broad concept of health and wellbeing with a version of client-centredness that permits them to engage in dialogue and negotiation with clients when the client's perspectives are at odds with the clinician's charter as a health professional. To position themselves appropriately in working with such clients, clinicians can draw upon multifaceted professional reasoning principles to help them support clients who seek to engage in occupations that are not commensurate with health, law, or societal standards.

References

American Occupational Therapy Association (2014). Occupational therapy practice framework: Domain and process (3rd ed.). *American Journal of Occupational Therapy*, 68(Suppl. 1), S1–S48. http://dx.doi.org/10.5014/ajot.2014.682006.

Aziz, M., & Sumaira, R. (2018). Risk taking behavior and interpersonal relationship of adrenaline junkies: A qualitative study. *Indian Journal of Health and Wellbeing*, 9(3), pp. 384–391.

Bersoff, D.M. (1999). Explaining unethical behaviour among people motivated to act prosocially. *Journal of Moral Education*, 28(4), pp. 413–428. https://doi.org/10.1080/030572499102981.

Boyt Schell, B.A. (2018). Pragmatic reasoning. In B.A. Boyt Schell & J.W. Schell (Eds.), *Clinical and professional reasoning in occupational therapy* (2nd ed.) (pp. 203–223). Philadelphia: Wolters Kluwer.

Boyt Schell, B.A., & Benfield, A. (2018). Aspects of professional reasoning. In B.A. Boyt Schell & J.W. Schell (Eds.), *Clinical and professional reasoning in occupational therapy* (2nd ed.) (pp. 127–144). Philadelphia: Wolters Kluwer.

Chapparo, C., & Ranka, J. (2000). Clinical reasoning in occupational therapy. In J. Higgs & M. Jones (Eds.), *Clinical reasoning in the health professions* (2nd ed.) (pp. 128–137). Oxford: Butterworth Heinemann.

Creek, J., & Hughes, A. (2008). Occupation and health: A review of selected literature. *British Journal of Occupational Therapy*, 71(11), pp. 456–468. https://doi.org/10.1177/030802260807101102.

Dodge, R., Daly, A., Huyton, J., & Sanders, L. (2012). The challenge of defining wellbeing. *International Journal of Wellbeing*, 2(3), pp. 222–235. https://doi. org/10.5502/ijw.v2i3.4.

Hamilton, T. (2018). Narrative reasoning. In B.A. Boyt Schell & J.W. Schell (Eds.), *Clinical and professional reasoning in occupational therapy* (2nd ed.) (pp. 171–202). Philadelphia: Wolters Kluwer.

Josef, A.K., Richter, D. Samanez-Larking, G.R., Wagner, G.G., Hertwig, R., & Mata, R. (2016). Stability and change in risk taking propensity across the lifespan. *Journal of Personality and Research Psychology*, 111(3), pp. 430–450. https://doi. org/10.1037/pspp.0000090.

Robertson, L., & Griffiths, S. (2012). Problem solving in occupational therapy. In L. Robertson (Ed.), *Clinical reasoning in occupational therapy: Controversies in practice* (pp. 1–14). Pondicherry: Wiley-Blackwell.

Slater, D.Y., Doherty, R.F., & Erler, K.S. (2018). Ethical reasoning. In B.A. Boyt Schell & J.W. Schell (Eds.), *Clinical and professional reasoning in occupational therapy* (2nd ed.) (pp. 225–244). Philadelphia: Wolters Kluwer.

Szumski, F., Bartels, R.M., Beech, A.R., & Fisher, D. (2018). Distorted cognition related to male sexual offending: The multi-mechanism theory of cognitive distortions (MMT-CD). *Aggression and Violent Behavior*, 39, pp. 139–151. https://doi. org/10.1016/j.avb.2018.02.001.

Tomlin, G.S. (2018). Scientific reasoning and evidence in practice. In B.A. Boyt Schell & J.W. Schell (Eds.), *Clinical and professional reasoning in occupational therapy* (2nd ed.) (pp. 145–169). Philadelphia: Wolters Kluwer.

Turpin, M.J., & Copley, J.A. (2018). Interactive reasoning. In B.A. Boyt Schell & J.W. Schell (Eds.), *Clinical and professional reasoning in occupational therapy* (2nd ed.) (pp. 245–260). Philadelphia: Wolters Kluwer.

Van Hoorn, J., Fuligini, A.J., Erone, E.A., & Galvan, A. (2016). Peer influence effects on risk taking and prosocial decision-making in adolescence. *Current Opinion in Behavioral Science*, 10, pp. 59–64. https://doi.org/10.1016/j.cobeha. 2016.05.007.

Weiss, N.H., Sullivan, T.P., & Tull, M.T. (2015). Explicating the role of emotion dysregulation in risky behaviors: A review and synthesis of the literature with directions for future research and clinical practice. *Current Opinion in Psychology*, 3, pp. 22–29. https://doi.org/10.1016/j.copsyc.2015.01.013.

World Health Organization (2001). *International classification of functioning, disability and health: ICF*. Geneva: World Health Organization.

World Health Organization (2002). *World report on violence and health*. Geneva: World Health Organization.

11 Substance use and recovery as part of daily life

A Zimbabwean perspective of substance use as an occupation among young adults living with HIV

Clement Nhunzvi and Roshan Galvaan

Introduction

Occupational therapy and occupational science should face the reality of challenging the taken for granted notion of a clear divide between "healthy" and "unhealthy" occupations if the field is to be true to its holistic and occupational philosophy. In doing so, experience and meaning pose as better yardsticks for exploring occupations. The potency of occupational narratives in capturing meaning of engagement in context is here emphasised.

Occupation is the core of occupational therapy and occupational science. True to this call, is the need for occupation-based practice, directed towards understanding how human occupation is initiated, actioned, and sustained, with its link to health and well-being (Lee, 2010). In this practice the use of occupation, as means and end, is emphasised on the assumptions that: there are occupations which are inherently health-promoting, occupation positively enables people to be self-sufficient, and occupation serves to be the primary organiser of time and resources (Yerxa, et al., 1990). Full understanding and application of occupation-based practice is only possible through the understanding of occupation in its entirety (Ward, Mitchell, & Price, 2007). However, despite being the core element in occupational therapy and occupational science, occupation remains a very complex phenomenon and complex to study and apply (Fogelberg & Frauwirth, 2010).

Occupation has long been known as an innate human need, which has the potential to address both the physical and mental health of an individual (Kuo, 2011). The overly positive and health-promoting nature of occupation has been challenged of late in a bid to be true to the holistic nature of occupational therapy. The traditionally unexplored occupations are coming to the fore and, interestingly, highlighting the need to understand them even in our quest to discourage participation in those occupations. From this position, it has been suggested that exploring the dark side of occupation can provide rich insight and direction in achieving a balanced, comprehensive, and inclusive view of human occupation (Twinley, 2013). At a time when the world is faced with a rise in self-damaging, deviant, or disruptive engagements, occupational science and occupational therapy can build on this and provide answers on the occupational nature of these engagements, thereby increasing its social relevance (Pierce, 2012). Voices of those engaging in these occupations are instrumental in capturing the experiential meaning of such engagements. Substance use is one such engagement that has remained under-explored from an occupational perspective (Nhunzvi, Galvaan, & Peters, 2017).

The following are some of the many benefits of occupations as framed in occupational therapy and occupational science, showing the need to explore beyond the assumed healthful nature of occupations:

- Occupations provide opportunities for individuals to experience flow, make contributions to themselves and others and discover meaning through action (Lee, 2010).
- For the output of occupation, all human systems are involved, hence the holistic nature of occupational therapy. When occupation is applied with wholeness, purpose and meaning in place of mere activities, it can also influence the client's psychological, emotional and social well-being (Ward, Mitchell, & Price, 2007).
- Engaging in occupations allows the person to achieve mastery in their environment. Through occupations, there is action on the environment and a response to environmental challenges (Kielhofner, 2008).
- Occupation is the doorway to understanding humans; this is because humans attach symbolic meaning to their occupations (Yerxa et al., 1990), and individuals and collectives are most true to their humanity when they engage in occupations.
- Occupation has the power to heal and is the main modality and unique contribution of occupational therapy to the health system (Kielhofner, 2004).
- To engage in occupations means to take control and this has economic, organisational and health implications. People can influence their health and society by their occupations (Wilcock, 2006).
- The configuration of occupations represents a balance which is optimal for health and this healthful balance of occupations in daily lives prevents incapacity (Yerxa et al., 1990).
- Occupation allows for the attainment of the major outcomes of occupational therapy, which are social and occupational participation (Ward, Mitchell, & Price, 2007).
- Participation in occupations leads to social participation and eventually social inclusion (Whiteford & Pereira, 2012).

Evidently, the understanding and application of occupation is broadening, with many occupational constructs emerging and being explored through research and practice, including: occupational choice (Galvaan, 2012), occupational consciousness (Ramugondo, 2015), and collective occupation (Fogelberg & Frauwirth, 2010; Ramugondo & Kronenberg, 2013), and many others related to occupational justice and injustice.

Occupational nature of substance use

Substance use knowledge continues to grow and become more complex; the field still warrants further exploration, especially from the service user's point of view (Cloud & Granfield, 2001; Helbig & McKay, 2003). The dominant discourses framing our knowledge and understanding of substance use are within medicine, criminality, morality, law, economics, politics, and popular culture. In occupational therapy and the general medical field, substance use has been problematised from the perspective of the well-known and commonly used disease model (Hyman, 2014). In dominant mental health literature, substance use is talked about more from the view of a disorder. The landmark publication, the DSM-V, spells out how largely psychoactive substances give rise to disorders. They present a case of substance use disorders, whereby the maladaptive pattern of substance use leads to clinically significant impairment or distress, shown by recurrent substance use leading to: failure in fulfilling major obligatory roles, engagement in physically hazardous situations, and recurrent legal problems or persistent social or interpersonal problems occurring over a 12-month period (DSM-V, American Psychiatric Association, 2013).

From the dominant discourses, consequences of substance use are diverse and range from biological to psychological and social areas of a person's life (Nordfjaern, Rundmo, & Hole, 2010). In occupational therapy, substance use is known to affect the body structure and function, thereby reducing occupational participation, which negatively affects health and quality of life. The occupational performance and identity areas of the user, the family, and society are all affected by substance abuse (Martin, Bliven, & Boisvert, 2008), making it a social problem. All these problems are further worsened by an unstable environment marked with stigma and discrimination. In South Africa, alcohol consumption by pregnant mothers has been conceptualised as both individualised and imposed occupation, where contextual forces weigh in on the mothers' occupational choices; alcohol consumption is, therefore, a survival occupation (Cloete & Ramugondo, 2015). This led us to question what substance use and abuse means to those who engage, despite its health-damaging nature, and whether there are benefits to this engagement.

Exploring substance abuse as an occupation among young adult Zimbabwean men

We carried out a narrative inquiry using an occupational perspective to explore the journey of recovery from substance abuse among young adult Zimbabwean men (see Nhunzvi et al., 2017). We purposively selected three young adult men who met the inclusion criteria to participate in in-depth narrative interviews about their occupations before and during recovery. Following the interviews, data were analysed using a narrative analysis. Explanatory stories and three superordinate themes illustrated how substance abuse was experienced as both an individual and a collective occupation associated with both positive and negative outcomes.

The stories shared by the participants suggested that substance abuse had become a central occupation prior to recovery. To them, substance abuse was experienced as an occupation shaping their health and well-being. Sense of belonging in a collective of like-minded young men, control, enjoyment of life, and stress relief were reported as their positive outcomes from substance abuse. They also said using the substances – even in risky situations – resonated with the traditional sociocultural belief and value system in most parts of Zimbabwe, where substance use was a marker of manhood and socialisation.

However, with continued and deepening substance use, health and social problems resulted. Two of the young men succumbed to substance-induced psychosis. The dominant biomedical approach and the criminalisation of substance use in Zimbabwe did not do much to help understand the experiential meaning of their engagements, and relapses were to characterise their recovery journeys.

Substance use also grew to be a central occupation around which other occupations were organised. The young men's meaningful use of time and energy resources was largely framed around substance use, also aiding their socialisation and developing an identity (Nhunzvi et al., 2017).

Addictions and impulse-control disorders have also been conceptualised as being occupational in nature (Kiepek & Magalhães, 2011). The young men who engaged in substance abuse associated abusing substances with gaining meaning in life and a feeling of subjective well-being. Hence occupational therapists and other mental health practitioners need to acknowledge alternative views in their management of substance use or abuse as engagements which can allow for the meaningful use of time and the development of meaning in life for those engaging in it (Nhunzvi et al., 2017; Wasmuth et al., 2014). Nevertheless, those "positive" outcomes are usually accompanied by the experience of "negative" consequences, including detrimental health effects and socially unacceptable behaviour (Chang, 2008; Kiepek & Magalhães, 2011; Nhunzvi et al., 2017; Twinley, 2013), indicating the complexity of substance use as an occupation. The use and abuse of substances, understood as an occupation in and of itself, might be a helpful way to conceptualise this phenomenon and the complexities associated with recovery.

In our study, we conceptualised recovery as an ongoing occupational transition: from the central occupation of substance use, and those occupations which sustained engagement in this, to a life dominated by "engaging occupations" which served to help the young adults in recovery to develop an identity of sobriety, health, and productive living (Nhunzvi et al., 2017). The men became more socially included in mainstream society, as they were accepted by their families and communities.

We found that occupations change over time. Occupational transition is not understood as continuity, but as a break with previous engagements, and as the building of new identities. Recovery is, therefore, better supported as a change process over time, negotiated through occupations for construction or reconstruction of an adaptive and "healthy" occupational identity. By understanding the occupational nature of substance use, and framing recovery as an occupational transition, occupational therapy is better positioned to be holistic. Hence the need to explore the environment shaping occupational choices and the recovery transition, rather than only seeing the occupation in isolation. This insight can better position occupational therapists to understand rather than judge occupations.

"Nicky":[1] a case of "risky" occupations for survival and inclusion in the context of HIV and substance use

Understanding under-explored occupations is paramount when working with people who engage in "risky" occupations for survival and inclusion, as the case scenario below demonstrates in the context of HIV and substance use. As questions around under-explored occupations like substance use continue to grow, it is time we regularly listened to and reported the voices of those experiencing it.

Nicky, who identifies as a lesbian, is a young adult living with HIV and is using substances – to survive and get a sense of inclusion against the full knowledge of negative consequences involved. In her reflections, Nicky shares a story where her solutions to her troubled life are actually the medical diagnosis she is being managed for.

> My name is Nicky, a Zimbabwean girl. I lost the soft and tender touch of a mother at a tender age. I was sexually abused by my own father; the abuse was to be followed by many abuses as I was navigating the unfriendly terrain of the world. I am living on the margins; I have found ways to keep me numb to the pain and have some sense of belonging as I seek survival and social inclusion. There is substance abuse, sex work, gangsterism, lesbianism, and illegal drug trade, structuring my days, giving meaning in life, and a sense of identity. I endure

stigma and discrimination, what they stigmatise keeps me going. My life will only make sense to you if you also use my eyes to see.

I was stressed, attempted suicide at 15, failing to comprehend what I was going through. No one would believe my version of the story. I was traumatised and was living together with my dad, so I decided to quench the pain through drugs. At least it was a journey with company, and I was beginning to find myself again. Although the substance abuse pushed me away and out of my family, it surely made me feel loved and belonging among my friends and compatriots.

I went deeper into substances and all that went with it. I joined a gang for protection and belonging. They made me sell drugs, I went into sex work, I was abused in the gang, sought protection in other gangs, but paid them by having sex with them. It went on and it became routine and habitual. I became tired of the abuse, it turned me off against all men, being abused by my father was weighing in. I found closure in same-sex relationships. Despite the illegality of same-sex practices in Zimbabwe, we risked all we had to, because that seemed to answer my desire to be loved without abuse. Along the way I contracted HIV, not that this changed much in my activities and engagements; it just added to the stigmatised identities I was already carrying. I have no sound education, I am not productively skilled, and there is no employment to talk of, and I am not a member of any church organisation. I live on the margins where I am socially included among people of my kind. What we do is necessary and makes the days go by. I have been through rehabilitation, it failed because it targeted one when we are many, a changed me is not sustainable when my circles and my spaces are not changed.

Nicky gets referred for occupational therapy. Where should the occupational therapist start? If occupation is everything people do which influences their health and well-being, impacting and impacted by their environments, occupational choices, and is the core of occupational therapy, then the dark side of occupation is a worthy concept for practice. In-depth exploration and experiential meaning of substance use, gangsterism, sex work, same-sex sex, and drug dealing as occupations are foundational to fully understand Nicky's occupational profile and needs. From there the well-informed occupational therapist can collaboratively work with all stakeholders to promote engagement in other, more socially inclusive occupations evidenced to promote recovery.

In delivering a truly holistic and occupation-centred service, we need to know how the traditionally segregated, criminalised, and largely health-damaging occupations seem to be answering to the human needs for participation and social inclusion. The nature of occupations versus the nature or patterns of engagement in those occupations stands as another area warranting exploration.

Ethical issues in being truly occupation-based in practice

Ethical issues are a notable and unavoidable part of occupational therapy practice across the globe. Contextual issues can minimise or complicate the uncertainties, distress, and dilemmas involved. Low resource settings and mental health practice areas are more complex than others. At the heart of occupational therapy practice is the issue of ethics, with the World Federation of Occupational Therapists (WFOT) asserting the call through its code of ethics (WFOT, 2016). There is a clear call to base ethical principles and values on the philosophical base of the profession, meaning the holistic nature of the approach, having occupation as the core of practice, and being truly person-centred. However, this seems so easy and doable without considering other occupations service users may be engaging in which are under-explored and judged to be overly health-damaging.

Under all circumstances an occupational therapist is expected to uphold traditional ethical principles and values. All humans have rights, including occupational rights (Hammell & Iwama, 2012), so the challenge presents when those rights need us to question the taken for granted and move out of our comfort zones. For instance, we are called on to abide by the laws governing our practice in context and at the same time not to discriminate against people based on race, colour, impairment, disability, national origin, age, gender, sexual preference, religion, political beliefs or status in society (WFOT, 2016).

As a case example, imagine being an occupational therapist in Zimbabwe, where the current laws criminalise same-sex relationships, meaning many people with diverse sexual and gender identities continue to face discrimination, harassment, intimidation, violence, blackmail, and prosecution – even at the hands of the state. Your service user is a victim of this. What do you address, and whose agenda do you serve? Next consider this: the WFOT (2016) code of ethics requires us to recognise that relatives/significant others are important, and to involve them. If the significant other of your service user happens to be their same-sex partner, do you recognise them in the land that does not recognise their relationship? Such ethical and sociolegal issues have remained in the dark and under-explored, meaning we are faced with a paucity of empirical evidence to guide ethical and evidence-based practice.

There are some difficult questions we need to ask ourselves and continue to reflect on as we begin to explore and apply knowledge generated through the concept of the dark side of occupation:

• Are we holistic and person-centred, when we play down under-explored occupations?
• When it comes to systemic and cultural ethical issues, are we using an occupational ethical lens or mere moral judgement about "unhealthy" occupations?

- When working with marginalised and stigmatised groups, to what extent do we uphold the collaborative goal setting approach, or are we reductionistic and prescriptive?
- When faced with the dark side of occupation, are we occupational and person-centred?
- Can we be of help on matters we don't understand – dealing with the under-explored occupations?
- How do we remain non-judgemental and help those who experience the world of occupations differently from us?
- Are all occupations the means and ends to health, well-being, and meaning? If not, is it because we know, or we lack understanding?

Conclusion

A call for holistic, ethical, evidence-based, occupation-centred and person-centred practice is recognised and furthered, as there is now the requirement to consider the concept of "the dark side of occupation" (Twinley, 2013). Substance use is one such occupation that has remained under-explored from an occupational perspective. However, there is a promising body of knowledge building which would help occupational therapists to better understand "healthy" and "unhealthy" occupations, and consequently holistically support occupational participation, health, well-being and social inclusion. In the process, the profession should brace-up for the ethical dilemmas accompanying this trajectory.

Note

1 Nicky (pseudonym) is one of the participants in the first author's doctoral study exploring an occupational perspective of social inclusion among young adults dually afflicted with substance use disorders and HIV in Zimbabwe. This work was supported through the DELTAS Africa Initiative [DEL-15-01]. The DELTAS Africa Initiative is an independent funding scheme of the African Academy of Sciences' (AAS) Alliance for Accelerating Excellence in Science in Africa (AESA) and supported by the New Partnership for Africa's Development Planning and Coordinating Agency (NEPAD Agency) with funding from the Wellcome Trust [DEL-15-01] and the UK government. The views expressed in this publication are those of the authors and not necessarily those of the AAS, the NEPAD Agency, the Wellcome Trust or the UK government.

References

American Psychiatric Association (2013). *Diagnostic and statistical manual of mental disorders (DSM-5®)*. (5th ed.). Arlington, VA: American Psychiatric Association.

Chang, E. (2008). Drug use as an occupation: Reflecting on Insite, Vancouver's supervised injection site. *Occupational Therapy Now*, 10(3), pp. 21–23.

Cloete, L.G., & Ramugondo, E.L. (2015). "I drink": Mothers' alcohol consumption as both individualised and imposed occupation. *South African Journal of Occupational Therapy, 45*(1), pp. 34–40. http://dx.doi.org/10.17159/2310-3833/2015/v45n1a6.

Cloud, W., & Granfield, R. (2001). Natural recovery from substance dependency: Lessons for treatment providers. *Journal of Social Work Practice in the Addictions, 1*, pp. 83–105. https://doi.org/10.1300/J160v01n01_07.

Fogelberg, D., & Frauwirth, S. (2010). A complexity science approach to occupation: Moving beyond the individual. *Journal of Occupational Science, 17*(3), pp. 131–139. doi:10.1080/14427591.2010.9686687.

Galvaan, R. (2012). Occupational choice: The significance of socio-economic and political factors. In G. Whiteford & C. Hocking (Eds.), *Occupational science: Society, inclusion, participation* (1st ed., pp. 152–162). Oxford: Blackwell Publishing.

Hammell, K.R.W., & Iwama, M.K. (2012). Well-being and occupational rights: An imperative for critical occupational therapy. *Scandinavian Journal of Occupational Therapy, 19*(5), pp. 385–394. doi:10.3109/11038128.2011.611821.

Helbig, K., & McKay, E. (2003). An exploration of addictive behaviours from an occupational perspective. *Journal of Occupational Science, 10*(3), pp. 140–145. https://doi.org/10.1080/14427591.2003.9686521.

Hyman, S.E. (2014). Addiction: A disease of learning and memory. *American Journal of Psychiatry, 162*(8), pp. 1414–1422. doi:10.1176/appi.ajp.162.8.1414.

Kielhofner, G. (2004). *Conceptual foundations of occupational therapy* (3rd ed.). Philadelphia: F.A. Davis Company.

Kielhofner, G. (2008). *Model of human occupation: Theory and application* (4th ed.). Baltimore: Williams & Wilkins.

Kiepek, N., & Magalhães, L. (2011). Addictions and impulse-control disorders as occupation: A selected literature review and synthesis. *Journal of Occupational Science, 18*(3), pp. 254–276. https://doi.org/10.1080/14427591.2011.581628.

Kuo, A. (2011). A transactional view: Occupation as a means to create experiences that matter. *Journal of Occupational Science, 18*(2), pp. 131–138.

Lee, J. (2010). Achieving best practice: A review of evidence linked to occupation-focused practice models. *Occupational Therapy in Health Care, 24*(3), pp. 206–223. https://doi.org/10.1080/14427591.2011.575759.

Martin, L.M., Bliven, M., & Boisvert, R. (2008). Occupational performance, self-esteem, and quality of life in substance addictions recovery. *Occupational Therapy Journal of Research, 28*(2), pp. 81–90. https://doi.org/10.3928/15394492-20080301-05.

Nhunzvi, C., Galvaan, R., & Peters, L. (2017). Recovery from Substance Abuse among Zimbabwean Men: An Occupational Transition. *OTJR: Occupation, Participation and Health, 39*(1), pp. 14–22. doi:10.1177/1539449217718503.

Nordfjaern, T., Rundmo, T., & Hole, R. (2010). Treatment and recovery as perceived by patients with substance addiction. *Journal of Psychiatric and Mental Health Nursing, 17*(1), pp. 46–64. doi:10.1111/j.1365-2850.2009.01477.x.

Pierce, D. (2012). Promise. *Journal of Occupational Science, 19*(4), pp. 298–311. doi:10.1080/14427591.2012.667778.

Ramugondo, E.L. (2015). Occupational consciousness. *Journal of Occupational Science, 22*(4), pp. 488–501. https://doi.org/10.1080/14427591.2015.1042516.

Ramugondo, E., & Kronenberg, F. (2013). Explaining collective occupations from a human relations perspective: Bridging the individual-collective dichotomy. *Journal of Occupational Science, 22*(1), pp. 3–16. doi:10.1080/14427591.2013.781920.

Twinley, R. (2013). The dark side of occupation: A concept for consideration. *Australian Occupational Therapy Journal, 60*(4), pp. 301–303. doi:10.1111/1440-1630. 12026.

Ward, K., Mitchell, J., & Price, P. (2007). Occupation-based practice and its relationship to social and occupational participation in adults with spinal cord injury. *OTJR: Occupation, Participation and Health, 27*(4), pp. 149–156. https://doi. org/10.1177/153944920702700405.

Wasmuth, S., Crabtree, J.L., & Scott, P.J. (2014). Exploring addiction-as-occupation. *British Journal of Occupational Therapy, 77*(12), pp. 605–613. doi:10.4276/030 802214X14176260335264.

Whiteford, G.E., & Pereira, R.B. (2012). Occupation, inclusion, participation. In G. Whiteford & C. Hocking (Eds.), *Occupational science: Society, inclusion, participation* (1st ed., pp. 185–207). Oxford: Blackwell Publishing.

Wilcock, A.A. (2006). *An occupational perspective of health.* Thorofare, NJ: Slack.

World Federation of Occupational Therapists (revised 2016). Code of ethics for occupational therapists. Retrieved from www.wfot.org/resources/code-of-ethics.

Yerxa, E.J., Clark, F., Frank, G., Jackson J., Parham, D., Pierce D., … Zemke, R. (1990). An introduction to occupational science: A foundation for occupational therapy in the 21st century. *Occupational Therapy in Health Care, 6*(4), pp. 1–17.

12 The dark side of occupation in an eating disorder intensive day service

Mary Cowan and Clarissa Sørlie

How we discovered the dark side of occupation

As a student in 2011, Clarissa attended Rebecca Twinley and Gareth Addi‑dle's presentation about the dark side of occupation at the "Owning Occupation" Occupational Science conference in Plymouth, UK. She continued to reflect on the concept throughout her final year of university, and in her first qualified role as an occupational therapist on a female acute mental health ward.

We – Mary and Clarissa – met in 2013, when Clarissa started working for an occupational therapy-led intensive day service for people with long-standing eating disorders. The programme seeks to understand individuals' subjective experience of their eating disorder and its impact on their everyday life, and to work with individuals towards their goals.

Mary was Clarissa's supervisor, and Clarissa shared her reflections on the application of the dark side of occupation in eating disorders during one of her supervision sessions. Being introduced to the concept of the dark side of occupation was a pivotal event in Mary's professional practice. The idea that occupations may not always be health-promoting, or indeed, the idea that illness behaviours (such as those behaviours that accompany eating disorders) could also be conceptualised as occupations in their own right, was, on reflection, something that she had given little consideration to. Shining the light on the dark side within her own practice involved a personal paradigm shift for Mary, both in her clinical reasoning, and in her understanding of occupation. One of the questions Mary grappled with was whether occupations were on the dark side because individuals chose to keep them hidden, or whether we as professionals prevented a discourse from taking place due to our own biases in how we view the construct of "occupation".

Exploring the dark side of occupation

Enthused by the possibilities that the concept afforded, we set out to develop a shared understanding of the dark side of occupation in eating disorders. Over the next few months, we pooled our collective knowledge of occupation, mental health, and eating disorders. We also sought new knowledge. For example, Clarissa researched pro-anorexia ("Pro-Ana") and pro-bulimia ("Pro-Mia") websites and had many conversations with Sarah Mercer (author of Chapter 8 in this text) about the function and meaning of occupations embedded within an eating disorder. We further refined our ideas during Skype calls with Rebecca Twinley, and through ongoing conversations with other eating disorder clinicians from a range of professional backgrounds. Throughout this process, we continued to reflect together about our developing thoughts on the topic, and the potential implications this would have for our practice.

Eating disorder behaviours as occupation

When we first began to apply the concept of the dark side of occupation to eating disorders, Elliot's (2012) paper on the "figured" – or lived – world of eating disorders was instrumental in shaping our thinking. Elliot argues that eating disorder behaviours (such as restricting, bingeing, and purging) could be defined as occupations. She acknowledges that "to make such a statement challenges the implicit assumption in the definition that meaning in occupation is health promoting and life-affirming" (Elliot, 2012, p. 17).

Elliot (2012) suggests that occupations exist on a continuum, with a "healthy, engaged experience of an occupation" (p. 17) on one end, and on the other, an occupational experience where previously neutral occupations have become "reinforced with illness-focused meaning" (p. 17). Elliot gives the following useful case example:

> In the figured world, Anne runs to purge calories, to distance herself from the onslaught of negative thoughts, to relieve her building anxiety, and because the loudest voice she hears is the one telling her that she "must" (Dignon, Beardsmore, Spain, & Kuan, 2006). It helps her feel special, taking satisfaction in her ability to do what others cannot (Weaver et al., 2005), which is to push her body past the point of exhaustion. Outside this figured world, running is a socially acceptable leisure pursuit offering multiple meanings depending on personal connection to this occupation (Primeau, 1996). In both lived worlds, the occupation of running and occupational identity as a runner appears similar. Yet in self-authoring, the conventional social discourse (healthy activity) and Anne's internal dialogue (punishment and escape) possess diametrically opposed meanings in how she navigates and participates in this single occupation.
>
> (Elliot, 2012, p. 19)

Writing about occupation and personality disorder, Jones (2010) similarly highlights the importance of understanding the meaning and motivation underlying occupations. She cautions that "superficial analysis may indicate that a client's engagement in occupation is adaptive when it is actually pathologically driven" (p. 204). We were therefore convinced that it was important not only to explore eating disorder-specific occupations but also to cultivate a sense of curiosity about the meaning and motivation underpinning participation in all occupations.

Starting conversations about the dark side of occupation

At the time that we considered explicitly introducing the concept of the dark side of occupation to our practice, we were already facilitating a weekly occupation-focused group called "Occupation Matters" (Sørlie & Cowan, 2015). The group had grown out of the foundations of the Lifestyle Redesign programme (Mandel, Jackson, Zemke, Nelson, & Clark, 1999), and drew heavily on Pierce's (2003) framework for therapeutic power. Discussion topics included occupational balance, occupational alienation, and meaning through occupation. Group participants had therefore been developing skills in occupational storytelling and occupational self-analysis (Craig & Mountain, 2006) for some time.

One week, we dedicated one session of the group to introducing the concept of the dark side of occupation and asked service users what they thought.

Their initial reaction: "It's a bit obvious, isn't it?"

But then they started sharing a range of experiences they had never spoken about in the group, and that we would not have thought to ask about. To respect the group's confidentiality boundaries, the detail of these experiences will not be recounted. However, we provide below a very broad overview of the themes that emerged.

We discussed as a group whether eating disorder behaviours (such as bingeing or over-exercising) could be considered "occupations". The answer was a resounding "yes". Individuals spoke about the meaning these behaviours held, how they gave structure to their day, and the goals often associated with them. Individuals acknowledged the discipline and effort that went into restriction and calorie-counting, and the sense of mastery and achievement that accompanied their "successful" efforts. Although these behaviours were surrounded by shame and secrecy, and individuals were aware that they were health-compromising, some of our service users also described experiencing them as compelling, appealing, satisfying, or even enjoyable.

In our experience, approaching the dark side of occupation with curiosity, and giving individuals permission to discuss their experiences in this way, opened up a more authentic dialogue about their lived experience. Using the label "the dark side of occupation" seemed to reduce some of the shame, fear, and secrecy surrounding discussions about the eating disorder.

Using the term also gave us a sense of being in a more objective space in which we could analyse the qualities of occupations on the dark side, and find other occupations that could meet similar needs. We reflected that there may previously have been an implicit expectation in the group that individuals should talk about wanting to give up their eating disorder – without enough validation of the value it held for the individual or how difficult that change would be. We found that using the language of "dark side" enabled group members, to some degree, to talk more openly about what they did in a way that did not "trigger" others. For example, some group members would choose to use the term "dark side" to refer to illness occupations, without giving more descriptive detail.

Our experience of these initial conversations convinced us that there was value in further applying the concept of the dark side of occupation to our practice. We were encouraged by how much sense the idea made to service users (to the extent that they would call it "obvious"), and by the shift we had noticed in conversations.

Impact on practice: occupational analysis

Given the sensitive nature of exploring occupations that have previously been hidden, our conversations about the dark side of occupation took place in the context of strong therapeutic relationships, robust clinical understanding of eating disorders, and a good grasp of therapeutic approaches, such as motivational interviewing. More often than not, this was done on an individual (rather than group) basis.

We approached these discussions as a collaborative exploration between equal partners. The service user could influence the pace and direction of the discussion, and we – the occupational therapists – had permission to ask questions and gently challenge.

Sessions were structured using the Daily Experiences of Pleasure, Productivity and Restoration Profile (Atler, 2014), now called the Occupational Experience Profile. This time-use diary provides a structure for individuals to reflect on their experience of occupations within a 24-hour timeframe. Individuals are asked to recount their time use in the previous day through discussion and reflection on what they did, when, and with whom. They are then asked to rate their experiences of pleasure, productivity and restoration on a 7-point rating scale. We already used Pierce's (2003) concepts of the subjective dimensions of occupation – productivity, pleasure, and restoration – in our Occupation Matters group, and service users were therefore well versed in the concepts.

Using this structure helped us to find out more about how our service users' days were organised, and where occupations they considered "on the dark side" fitted into their routines. We gently asked exploratory questions, particularly when our clinical knowledge and experience suggested that there might be omissions in an individual's account of their day.

These explorations often paved the way for conversations about what change would mean for the individual and the potential impact of the loss of eating disorder occupations. This helped us as clinicians to gain a deeper understanding of what we were asking of people each time we challenged their eating disorder. This understanding also gave us a foundation for exploring potential ways of filling the void left by the eating disorder with other, more health-promoting occupations. Our therapeutic relationships with service users grew stronger, the more that they felt we understood and respected their lived experience.

Service users reflected that they often felt misunderstood by professionals (including occupational therapists), particularly when interventions were focused on skill and performance. By increasing our awareness of meaning and motivation, we were able to work together with individuals to design individualised, meaningful interventions. We used the concepts of "occupational performance", "occupational understanding", or "occupational disposition" (Park, 2014) in our discussions and documentation to clarify what we were addressing. More often than not, our work on the dark side of occupation was focused on disposition (how someone feels about engaging in occupations).

Discussions about the dark side of occupation often led to conversations about secrecy. Individuals described having a "double life" in which they engage in covert activities, hidden from others. This was often associated with strong feelings of shame and fear. However, for some individuals, this secrecy – and the lengths they would go to in order to avoid detection – held a lot of meaning and value. There are many reasons why this is the case, and as always, it is highly individualised. For example, they may provide an individual with a way of doing something entirely for themselves, when they usually prioritise the needs of others, referred to as "Me Time". It may feel liberating to do something that is kept secret from others. And for some people, the risk of getting "caught" can provide a thrill or "buzz". By exploring this with individuals, we were able to work with them to identify other occupations that would meet similar needs.

The complexity of the notion of occupational balance became increasingly apparent when we began to acknowledge the conflicting demands of engaging in occupations service users perceived were "on the dark side", whilst also attempting to meet obligations, responsibilities, and expectations associated with relationships or productive life roles. This balance took a significant amount of mental and physical effort, and individuals described the demands they experienced from their eating disorder. The conflict between different spheres of life prompted individuals to reflect on what it would mean to lose illness behaviours from their repertoire of everyday habits and routines; therefore, highlighting the links between occupation and identity formation and development.

We first realised how firmly the concept of the dark side of occupation had become embedded in our service when one of our students on placement returned from an initial interview to ask us what the term "the dark side of occupation" meant. She explained that the individual she interviewed had spoken at length about it, and when the student mentioned that she had never heard the term before, the service user replied, "it's a pretty self-explanatory term, all occupational therapists should know it".

Context-relevant assessment and intervention

In our existing service model, most of our interventions took place in the hospital environment where service users attended the day service. The more we discussed the impact of context and environment (in its broadest sense) with service users, the more we became convinced that our work on the dark side of occupation needed to take place in individuals' own environments.

It was clear from our discussions that routines are mapped onto spaces and objects in the environment (Pierce, 2003), and that this is no different when it comes to the dark side of occupation. Elliot (2012) describes how otherwise neutral objects or behaviour can take on symbolic meaning through repeated use. For example, Elliot (2012) gives examples of a weighing scale becoming "the instrument against which ... self-worth is measured" (p. 19) and a bathroom at work becoming associated with purging.

Clarissa began to schedule visits with service users to their own homes, local cafés, restaurants, supermarkets, and even colleges/universities. Because this involved entering into individuals' personal spaces and social environments, Clarissa had detailed conversations with individuals beforehand about their own boundaries, preferences, and anxieties. For example, she negotiated with service users how she would introduce herself to their acquaintances or children (particularly when they were not aware that the service user was accessing treatment), how she might challenge eating disorder behaviours if others were present, or whether there were any spaces that the individual did not feel ready to show the occupational therapist. These boundaries constantly evolved throughout the work, and were therefore reviewed after each visit.

Clarissa accompanied individuals through their daily routines and engaged in a curious, open dialogue with them about what they would usually be doing. These visits yielded rich insights into the impact of the environment on the dark side of occupation. Many of these discoveries were new, not only to Clarissa, but also to the individual she was working with. The following day, she would meet with the individual to explore the learning that had arisen from the visit, including any reflections about the meaning of the dark side of occupation. She supported the individual to collaboratively analyse their habituation and environment and identify alternatives to the familiar patterns of the dark side of occupation. Some individuals found it helpful to use photographs of their environments (e.g. kitchens, bathrooms and bedrooms) as visual aids to refer to during these analyses, and also as a means of tracking changes post-intervention. Clarissa also drew on her training in Cognitive Analytic Therapy to incorporate circular diagrams into these discussions. They then scheduled follow-up visits to practise the changes they had identified (with graded support), with the aim of establishing new routines that fitted with the individual's goals. By the time she left the service, the majority of Clarissa's work took place in these environments.

Concluding remarks

Our experience of sharing the theory of the dark side of occupation with service users, and developing interventions in collaboration with them, has been powerful. For our service users, the combination of exploratory discussions and context-specific assessments and interventions introduced them to tools they could use to "become their own occupational therapist". It also gave individuals opportunities to develop a robust understanding of their own occupational lives, of the dark side of occupation and what it meant to them. For us as clinicians, it improved our relationships with service users, strengthened our clinical reasoning, and improved our satisfaction with our work.

We are not the first eating disorders clinicians to explore the dark side of occupation in eating disorders. However, we have shared our story here in the hope that it will be useful to you in your own journey with the concept. We invite you to continue to refine the idea, deepen the exploration, and share your reflections and findings, so we can build a more robust body of work together.

References

Atler, K.E. (2014). The Daily Experiences of Pleasure, Productivity and Restoration Profile. In D. Pierce (Ed.), *Occupational science for occupational therapy* (pp. 187–199). Thorofare, NJ: Slack.

Craig, C., & Mountain, G. (2006). *Lifestyle matters: An occupational approach to healthy ageing*. London: Routledge.

Elliot, M.L. (2012). Figured world of eating disorders: Occupations of illness. *Canadian Journal of Occupational Therapy*, *79*(1), pp. 15–22. doi:10.2182/cjot.2012. 79.1.3.

Jones, L. (2010). The role of the occupational therapist in treating people with personality disorder. In N. Murphy & D. McVey (Eds.), *Treating personality disorder: Creating robust services for people with complex mental health needs* (pp. 201–218). London: Routledge.

Mandel, D.R., Jackson, J.M., Zemke, R., Nelson, L., & Clark, F.A. (1999). *Lifestyle redesign: Implementing the well elderly program*. Bethesda, MD: AOTA Press.

Park, S. (2014). Outcome evaluation and documentation process in occupational therapy: Occupation-based, client-centered and context-relevant. Harrison Training.

Pierce, D. (2003). *Occupation by design: Building therapeutic power*. Philadelphia, PA: F.A. Davis Company.

Sørlie, C., & Cowan, M. (2015, June). Making occupation matter in an intensive eating disorder service. Paper presented at the College of Occupational Therapists 39th Annual Conference, Brighton, UK. doi:10.1177/0308022615583236.

Twinley, R., & Addidle, G. (2011, September). Anti-social occupations: Considering the dark side of occupation. Paper presented at the International Occupational Science Conference: Occupational Therapists Owning Occupation, Plymouth University, UK.

13 Occupational engagement in forensic settings

Exploring the occupational experiences of men living within a forensic mental health unit

Karen Morris

Background and introduction

I intend for this chapter to illuminate how I explored occupational engagement for men living in a regional secure mental health unit in the United Kingdom (UK). First, I briefly outline forensic mental health services in the UK before exploring the development of a new framework to explore the concept of occupational engagement within this setting. I then explore the relationship between occupational engagement and the dark side of occupation for both residents and staff working in forensic settings.

This research formed my PhD studies (see Morris, 2012). The starting point for this was a nagging question – how do we, as occupational therapists, *know* that the activities we offer as part of our assessment and intervention have value and meaning to the people we work with, especially in long-term settings? Other questions that are at the heart of the issues I explore within this chapter were:

- Just because something has value at the beginning of someone's stay in a unit, how often is this re-evaluated?
- What if the occupations that have most value to a person are not socially acceptable and therefore forbidden?
- What is the impact of this on occupational therapy practice within such settings?

Just as other contributors to this text have discussed and posed, at this point I would like to ask the reader to remind themselves of the difference between the "dark side" and "dark" occupations. The general dictionary definition of "dark" as having little or no light aligns with Twinley's

(2013) explanation of her concept that "occupation is something that has aspects which are less acknowledged, less explored and less understood. It presents occupation as something which has aspects to it that have been left in the shadows" (p. 302). Then, there is the understanding of "dark" or "dark side" as something (or someone) who is mysterious or secret, evil or threatening. Employing this latter interpretation, there is no doubt that some of the occupations residents in secure units have experienced are "dark", yet personal judgements about these need to be suspended to enable a full understanding of why people do the things they do – all occupations have illuminated and dark sides, whether socially acceptable or not.

The setting

Within a single chapter, it is not possible to explain all the intricacies of the UK forensic mental health system, but a very brief outline is hopefully useful to aid understanding if you are not familiar with this area. The UK has a community-focused mental health system with only about 6% of people admitted to hospital for treatment (CQC, 2009). Forensic mental health practitioners work within general mental health (inpatient, community, and supported accommodation settings), secure mental health, and prison services. Within the secure services, security levels are defined as high, medium, and low. In addition to this, there are specialist community teams and supported accommodation. There are around 6,000 secure inpatient beds (approximately: 680 high; 2,800 medium; 2,500 low security (JCPMH, 2013)). Of these people, 8/10 are men, with an average stay of 5–10 years (Rutherford & Duggan, 2008). As far as possible, people are held at the lowest level of security required for safety. If you would like to find out more about UK mental health services, please search for and access the guidance document by the Joint Commissioning Panel for Mental Health (2013).

Forensic mental health is a unique setting in that there are two clear purposes: (1) treating the person with mental illness, and (2) protection of society. The majority of residents are "involuntary", being detained under the Mental Health Act (2007). Another unique feature is that services do not have full autonomy with decisions; the Ministry of Justice can influence treatment as permission is often needed to change a person's security status, thereby impacting on their recovery journey, positive risk-taking and movement within areas (Centre for Mental Health, 2011). Successful treatment is first measured by reduction of symptoms and public safety before personal wellbeing (JCPMH, 2013). In recent years, as in other mental health areas, there has been an active focus on implementing recovery-oriented principles through use of the "My Shared Pathway" initiative (Livingston, 2018; Recovery & Outcomes, 2018). This has highlighted the tensions, and potential for conflict, between the two "masters" within forensic mental health services – the person and society. This is a significant culture shift which is beginning to be explored within the literature.

Forensic mental health is a growing area of practice for occupational therapy with active research contributions. In the UK, this emerging evidence base has been used to develop the National Institute for Health and Care Excellence (NICE) accredited practice guidelines (RCOT, 2017) to support therapists working with people living in secure hospitals. The impact of the additional restrictions from an occupational perspective are being explored, mainly through qualitative research (e.g. Alred, 2018; Cronin-Davis, 2010; Morris, 2012). This is ensuring that the voices of the people occupational therapists work with within these services remain strong. Additionally, the reflective nature of the methodologies used (e.g. action research, interpretative phenomenological analysis, social constructionism) are ensuring that researchers are also challenging the profession's long-held philosophical assumptions of the positive meaning of occupations to people (Hammell, 2009).

Exploring occupational engagement

My PhD research aimed to explore how the value of occupation changed over time for a small group of men living in a regional secure unit. Five men agreed to take part in the research and were interviewed four times over a year. In addition, I used participant observations and a review of their clinical notes to inform our conversations about how the value of their occupations changed during the year. I utilised a social constructionist methodology (Burr, 2003) and heuristic analysis (Moustakas, 1990). This approach enabled me to listen to the men's stories as a researcher, rather than a clinician, challenging my beliefs and understanding about the value and meaning of occupation in unexpected ways.

As already mentioned, within occupational therapy core texts, occupation traditionally has been assumed to be positive for health. For example, Duncan (2006, p. 30) said:

> Occupation has a central role in human life. It provides motive and meaning to life; lack of access to occupations may have a negative effect on health and quality of life; the use of occupation to address impacts on health or quality of life is the core of occupational therapy … Respect for the value of human life; the importance of individual empowerment and engagement in occupation; the integration of individuals into life through meaningful occupation.

The term "occupational engagement" has been frequently used within occupational therapy and occupational science literature, but without a consistent definition or use. Mary Reilly (1962) is often quoted as the source of the term, but it does not appear within the text cited. What she actually said was: "That man, though the use of his hands, as they are ener-gised by mind and will, can influence the state of his own health" (p. 2) – often quoted as the occupational therapy philosophy – but she went on to say: "This is the inherited occupational therapy *hypothesis passed on for proof* by the early founders" (p. 2, emphasis added) and "In our forty years of practice we have accumulated some *fascinating odds and ends of under-standing* about the need to work" (p. 4, emphasis added). So, what is often quoted as a statement, is actually a challenge to the profession.

The "creative synthesis" (Moustakas, 1990) of my research, rather than a simple definition of the term, was a new framework positioning occupa-tional engagement within a range of positive and negative values and consequences (see Figure 13.1 below). During the development of the framework, I held only the traditional view of my profession and initially only focused on the positive values of occupation. As the data analysis increased in depth, I was able to challenge this perspective and also explore the potential for negative value within occupations.

As illustrated, the framework considers the values and consequences of an occupation. Occupation is defined as a unique, one-off experience of an activity (Pierce, 2001). Occupational engagement is a fluctuating state influ-enced by complex and multiple factors. Occupational engagement is posi-tioned within a framework of personal value and perceived consequences

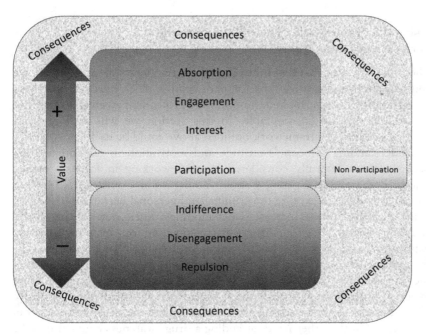

Figure 13.1 Framework to position occupational engagement.
Source: Morris, 2012; Morris & Cox, 2017.

to participation. Every occupation has a level of personal value, but also has consequences in terms of feedback from physical, social, and cultural environments. "Participation" is the anchor and entry point into the framework. Levels of value are represented as a continuum, from "absorption" as the most positive level of value, to "repulsion" as the most negative level. "Absorption", "Engagement" and "Interest" represent graded levels of positive value. So, "engaging" occupations require more involvement than those that just "interest" the individual, but not as much as "absorbing" occupations. On the other end of the scale, "Indifference", "Disengagement" and "Repulsion" represent graded levels of negative value.

It should be noted that "Non-Participation" is not considered to be occupation, as the definition of "occupation" used requires "doing" (i.e. active participation). However, non-participation is important and must be remembered as it serves a purpose; for example, it may be the only way that individuals have of controlling their environment. As well as value, the person will perceive positive or negative consequences to participation, which may change over time in response to feedback from their environment. An occupation with positive value for the individual can have negative consequences and vice versa. The aim of treatment within forensic settings is for people to participate in occupations with both positive personal value and positive perceived consequences for both the individual and society.

Using this framework to help illuminate the dark side of occupations

The framework may be helpful to illuminate the dark side of occupations, and to understand motivations for participating in occupations that have been traditionally overlooked, no doubt due to being perceived as negative or troublesome or unacceptable. In this section we will explore some examples of how the framework outlined above could be useful.

Understanding someone's attitude and motivation in relation to their occupations is carefully considered by staff working in forensic mental health. For example, Spruin, Canter, Youngs, and Coulston (2014) used narrative analysis to explore the criminal and personal narratives of 70 men living in secure units to increase understanding of their views of themselves and their crimes. They found that participants used four main narratives to explain their behaviour – hero, victim, professional, and revenger. The framework may support this exploration of why people do the things that they do (Morris, Cox, & Ward, 2016). For instance, taking illegal drugs might stimulate occupational interest or engagement (so therefore positive value) but can result in getting arrested (and therefore negative social consequence). On the other hand, attending a drug awareness course might be accompanied by occupational indifference (classed as negative value), motivated by increasing leave out of a unit, but can result in increased ability to manage without drugs (and therefore assumed positive consequence for the individual and society). Another example came to light when a clinician used the framework to structure a conversation with a resident about their poor personal care (Morris & Ward, 2018). The resident's refusal to shower was assumed to be about poor personal care (a common feature of his illness), but in reality, the water often went cold so showering was very unpleasant and no longer had positive consequences for him.

The emphasis within forensic mental health units is on relational and procedural security as much as physical security (JCPMH, 2013), but this does not fully alleviate the impact of restrictions. As in any setting, staff can quickly become desensitised to the impact of the work environment and the impact this can have on wellbeing. Healthcare professionals traditionally focus on the positive aspects of the impact of our interventions with an expectation of "first, do no harm". As already discussed, attitude and motivation are closely examined. Residents may be required to attend certain therapeutic groups before being eligible for increased leave from the unit, or discharge. It can be incredibly hard for clinicians to really hear some of the messages that they are given by residents in secure units. For example, we can all appreciate that it is not nice to have our movements and activities restricted by others, but it is easier for clinicians to focus on the potential positive therapeutic benefits of the unit rather than dwelling too much on the potential negative impact of the secure environment; as one of my research participants, Dave, reinforced when he asked "Am I your only torture victim today?" This was a man who hated living communally, but was not yet deemed "well enough" to move to a quieter part of the unit; for him the "therapeutic" environment within the unit was – as he expressed – "torture", only relieved with short periods of unescorted leave within the wider hospital grounds. This led Dave to be labelled as uncooperative when he expressed his frustrations (sometimes aggressively). Due to legal restrictions and the need to serve both masters (society as well as the individual), staff were unable to change the situation, sometimes leading to Dave feeling not listened to. The framework above could be used to support conversations to both understand the impact of the unit on Dave, but also to help Dave explore the dark side of his own occupations on his therapeutic journey.

Summary and key points

I echo Nastasi's (Chapter 17) assertion that analysing the impact of the environment on a person's subjective experience of occupation is crucial; environments such as secure mental health units add an additional layer of complexity to the exploration of the dark side of occupations. Theory, including the framework I have discussed within this chapter, is emerging that enables practitioners to fully explore the negative values and/or consequences of someone's occupations. I believe that occupational therapists can use this framework to help illuminate the dark side of occupations in a number of ways, for example:

- Using the framework to help structure conversations exploring both positive and negative aspects of occupations, illuminating why people do the things that they do (or no longer do).
- Using the framework as a reflective supervision tool to illuminate and explore the complex nature of occupations used within therapeutic interventions.
- Using the framework to help illuminate the impact of physical, social and cultural environments on occupations.

References

Alred, D. (2018). Service user perspectives of preparation for living in the community following discharge from a secure mental health unit (Doctoral dissertation, University of Brighton, UK). Retrieved from https://research.brighton.ac.uk/en/studentTheses/service-user-perspectives-of-preparation-for-living-in-the-commun.

Burr, V. (2003). *Social constructionism*. London and New York: Routledge.

Centre for Mental Health (2011). *Pathways to unlocking secure mental health care*. London: Centre for Mental Health Care.

CQC (2009). Patient survey report 2009: Mental health acute inpatient service users survey 2009. Retrieved from www.nhssurveys.org/Filestore/documents/MH09_RTQ.pdf.

Cronin-Davis, J. (2010). Occupational therapy practice with male patients diagnosed with personality disorder in forensic settings: A qualitative study of the views and perceptions of patients, managers and occupational therapists (Doctoral dissertation, University of Leeds, UK). Retrieved from https://ethos.bl.uk/OrderDetails.do?uin=uk.bl.ethos.699798.

Duncan, E.A.S. (2006). *Foundations for practice in occupational therapy* (4th ed.). Edinburgh: Churchill Livingstone Elsevier.

Hammell, K.W. (2009). Sacred texts: A sceptical exploration of the assumptions underpinning theories of occupation. *Canadian Journal of Occupational Therapy*, 76(1), pp. 6–22. doi:10.1177/000841740907600105.

Joint Commissioning Panel for Mental Health (JCPMH) (2013). Guidance for commissioners of forensic mental health services. Retrieved from www.jcpmh.info/wp-content/uploads/jcpmh-forensic-guide.pdf.

Livingston, J.D. (2018). What does success look like in the forensic mental health system? Perspectives of service users and service providers. *International Journal of Offender Therapy and Comparative Criminology*, 62(1), pp. 208–228. https://doi.org/10.1177/0306624X16639973.

Mental Health Act, 2007 (C 12). London: The Stationary Office.

Morris, K. (2012). Occupational engagement in a regional secure unit (Unpublished doctoral dissertation, Lancaster University, UK).

Morris, K., & Cox, D.L. (2017). Developing a descriptive framework for "occupational engagement". *Journal of Occupational Science*, 24(2), pp. 152–164. https://doi.org/10.1080/14427591.2017.1319292.

Morris, K., Cox, D.L., & Ward, K. (2016). Exploring stories of occupational engagement in a regional secure unit. *The Journal of Forensic Psychiatry & Psychology*, 27(5), pp. 684–697. https://doi.org/10.1080/14789949.2016.1187759.

Morris, K., & Ward, K. (2018). The implementation of a new conceptual framework for occupational engagement in forensic settings: Feasibility and application to occupational therapy practice. *Mental Health Review Journal*, 23(4), pp. 308–319. https://doi.org/10.1108/MHRJ-03-2018-0007.

Moustakas, C. (1990). *Heuristic research: Design, methodology and application*. London: Sage.

Pierce, D. (2001). Untangling occupation and activity. *The American Journal of Occupational Therapy*, 55(2), pp. 138–146. https://doi.org/10.5014/ajot.55.2.138.

Recovery & Outcomes (2018). My Shared Pathway. Retrieved from www.recoveryand outcomes.org/my-shared-pathway/my-shared-pathway.html.

Reilly, M. (1962). Occupational therapy can be one of the great ideas of 20th century medicine: The Eleanor Clarke Slagle Lecture. *The American Journal of Occupational Therapy*, 16(1), pp. 1–9.

Royal College of Occupational Therapists (RCOT) (2017). *Occupational therapists' use of occupation-focused practice in secure hospitals. Practice guideline* (2nd ed.). London: Royal College of Occupational Therapists.

Rutherford, M., and Duggan, S. (2008). Forensic mental health services: Facts and figures on current provision, *The British Journal of Forensic Practice*, 10(4), pp. 4–10. https://doi.org/10.1108/14636646200800020.

Spruin, E., Canter, D., Youngs D., & Coulston, B. (2014). Criminal narratives of mentally disordered offenders: An exploratory study. *Journal of Forensic Psychology Practice*, 14(5), pp. 438–455. https://doi.org/10.1080/15228932.2014.965987.

Twinley, R. (2013). The dark side of occupation: A concept for consideration. *Australian Occupational Therapy Journal*, 60(4), pp. 301–303. doi:10.1111/1440-1630. 12026.

14 The development of an assessment which provides a practical application of the concept of the dark side of occupation for practitioners and students

Quinn Tyminski

Introduction

Participation in the dark side of occupation occurs for all individuals in a variety of populations, contexts, and environments (Twinley, 2013). Yet, the prevalence of these occupations in some practice settings requires the development of valid assessment tools to accurately measure participation in all occupations, including the dark side of occupation (Tyminski et al., 2020). It is necessary to explore a holistic view of an individual's occupational participation to understand the entire person as an occupational being and prioritise interventions to increase independence around an individual's readiness to change.

Translational research

As a developing concept, the majority of the work regarding the dark side of occupation has focused largely on theoretical discussion, with Twinley (2017) calling for this to next be incorporated into education, practice, and research. Translational research moves the concept on to its practical application and implications. Originating from the field of oncology, translational science is relatively new, first appearing in the literature in 1993 (Westfall, Mold, & Fagnan, 2007). The definition of translational research utilised in the development of the ACS-AIP assessment is: "research aimed at adoption of best practice in the community" (Rubio et al., 2010, p. 3). Translational research in occupational therapy rapidly implements research findings into an array of practice settings to increase overall health, wellness, and health-related quality of life (Titler, 2018).

Many models, theories, and frameworks serve as a guide for translating research into practice, the most commonly used being the Diffusions of Innovations Theory (Rogers, 1995). In this theory, Rogers discussed the importance of diffusion, or the process through which a novel concept spreads amongst the members of a community of practice and innovation. In subsequent articles, Rogers presented numerous strategies for increasing the diffusion of innovations, among them the use of advocacy, social networks, and changing of the systematic norms (Rogers, 2002).

In the field of occupational therapy, the profession has long recognised the need for the transfer of knowledge between occupational science and occupational therapy (Clark et al., 1991). Occupational science is defined as the study of occupation (Yerxa et al., 1989). Occupational science differs from the field of occupational therapy, focusing on the basic science behind occupation rather than enabling participation. Yet, the field of occupational therapy can glean great insight from innovative concepts and theories of occupational science (Sainburg, Liew, Frey, & Clark, 2017). Thus, it is necessary to explore strategies for interpreting and applying occupational science work to evidence-based practice techniques that may be used by occupational therapy practitioners.

Further conceptualising the need for translational science in occupational therapy to the dark side of occupation, the theoretical concept of the dark side of occupation must be brought to the attention of occupational therapy practitioners in a tangible way, in order to secure its inclusion in the field of occupational therapy (Aldrich, Rudman, & Dickie, 2017; Townsend & Wilcock, 2004). Thus, an evidence-based assessment, which includes many of the occupations considered to be currently "in the dark", is necessary for occupational therapy practitioners. The Activity Card Sort-Advancing Inclusive Participation, a version of the evidence-based Activity Card Sort (Baum & Edwards, 2008), translates the dark side of occupation into a practical tool for clinicians looking to holistically evaluate their clients.

Development of the Activity Card Sort-Advancing Inclusive Participation

Originally designed for use with community-dwelling older adults, the Activity Card Sort (ACS) informs therapy goals by identifying changes in occupational participation (Baum & Edwards, 2008). It features 89 photographs, with captions, of adults engaged in occupations. The client sorts the cards into categories based on current and previous participation in each occupation. Yet, the activities depicted in previous iterations do not include many occupations that may be central to the lives of those who are homeless (Tyminski et al., 2020).

The profession of occupational therapy continues to call for greater inclusion of individuals, occupations, and environments (Kinebanian & Stomph, 2010). The need for a more inclusive assessment tool in the homeless population resulted in the development of a new version of the ACS, designed to capture the unique occupational participation of this population. Titled the Activity Card Sort-Advancing Inclusive Participation (ACS-AIP), this assessment tool provides a more inclusive view of occupational participation and promotes greater cultural inclusivity (Tyminski et al., 2020).

The ACS-AIP consists of 76 occupations depicted in line drawings with follow-up questions. It consists of occupations taken from the original version of the ACS, other occupations known to be participated in by the homeless population, and purposeful inclusion of the dark side of occupation. The ACS-AIP drew on literature, content expert feedback, and input of individuals experiencing homelessness to select these 76 occupations. In order to create an assessment with greater inclusivity, line drawings were selected to depict occupational participation on each card (see Figure 14.1). Further, line drawings on each card were manipulated to remove many identifying physical features representative of gender, race or culture, to create images of greater inclusivity. Finally, on the back of each card, follow-up questions were included to guide practitioners in deepening conversation related to participation in each occupation. Follow-up questions were included from a variety of sources including expert opinion, literature sources, and individuals experiencing homelessness request. The follow-up questions provide a guide for discussion surrounding difficult topics or

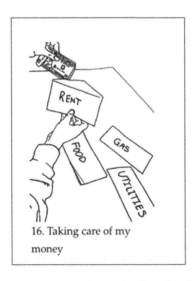
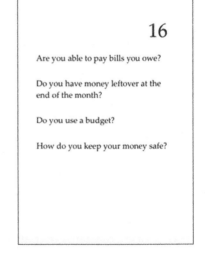

Figure 14.1 ACS-AIP Card # 16 and follow-up questions.

Source: Tyminski et al., 2020.

occupations, bridging the gap between the lived experience of the practitioner and the client (Tyminski et al., 2020).

Case study of the ACS-AIP: "John"

Consider the idea of assessing for an inclusive understanding of occupational participation by examining the case study of "John". John is a 21-year-old Caucasian male currently seeking services at a homeless services agency. During his semi-structured intake evaluation, John reveals he has been homeless for five years after being disowned by his family for self-identifying as gay. John reports a mental health diagnosis of severe depression and co-occurring substance use of cocaine. When asked about his ability to participate in his daily life, John reports "being homeless isn't the best – but I get along fine".

In order to glean greater information about John's occupational participation, the occupational therapy practitioner decides to administer the ACS-AIP to John. John sorted the 76 cards, each depicting a different occupation, into three piles, based on how often he participated in each item: "do now", "used to do", and "never did". Through the use of the ACS-AIP, John identified decreased participation in social, instrumental activities of daily living, and leisure occupations. John reported current participation in activities of daily living, resource seeking, and coping skills (see Table 14.1).

After John completed sorting the cards, the occupational therapy practitioner encouraged John to complete a secondary sort. John took all of the occupations sorted into the "used to do" pile and placed the occupations that he was interested in participating in into the new category of "want to do". John identified attending school, finding a romantic partner, dealing with legal issues, going to support groups, and managing his mail as desired occupations.

Based on the secondary sort, the occupational therapy practitioner can develop a treatment plan for John. For further information on John's occupational performance and participation, the practitioner has two options. First, the practitioner may select, at any point during the evaluation process, to utilise the questions on the back of each card. The follow-up questions guide the practitioner to deepen the conversation surrounding each occupation. For John, the occupational therapy practitioner may decide to ask follow-up questions regarding his previous identified occupations to determine the barriers to completing each occupation. This information supports the practitioner in determining how best to provide intervention with this client. Second, the practitioner may decide to use the occupational performance and satisfaction rating scale. In this case, the practitioner asks John to rank each occupation on his ability to perform the occupation and his satisfaction with his current level of performance (see Figure 14.2) (Baum, 2019). This is similar to the ranking that occurs during the Canadian Occupational Performance Measure, helping to track outcomes and identify treatment priorities (Law et al., 1990).

Table 14.1 John's occupational participation as reported by the ACS-AIP

Do now	Used to do	Never did
Dealing with stress and emotions	Applying for school	Biking
Eating	Attending school/classes	Dancing
Eating with others	Being in a relationship with a spouse or partner	Drawing art
Finding drugs/alcohol	Caring for loved ones who are ill	Gambling
Finding and using resources	Dealing with legal issues	Gardening
Finding clothing	Doing laundry	Managing pregnancy
Finding housing	Drinking alcohol	Overcoming addiction
Getting dressed	Driving	Playing sports
Getting hygiene items	Exercising	Taking care of feminine hygiene
Getting money	Taking out the trash	Taking care of my money
Going to gatherings	Going to public events	Taking pictures
Going to health appointments	Going to support groups	Using a computer
Going to place of worship	Going to the store	
Going to the beauty shop/ barbershop	Making music	
Going to the ER	Making something to eat	
Helping other people	Managing mail	
Journalling	Pursuing sex	
Keeping my living space clean	Spending time with friends	
Watching TV/movies	Taking care of a pet	
Working for pay/volunteering	Getting food and beverage	
Using public transit	Washing dishes	
Listening to music		
Looking for jobs		
Managing medications		
Playing tabletop games		
Praying		
Preventing pregnancy and infection		
Protecting my things		
Reading		
Seeking services		
Setting goals		
Sitting and thinking		
Sleeping		
Smoking cigarettes		
Spending time outside		
Stealing		
Taking care of family		
Taking care of myself & my hygiene		
Travelling		
Using a phone		
Using or misusing drugs		
Visiting public spaces (i.e. gardens, parks, museums, library)		

Activity One: _____

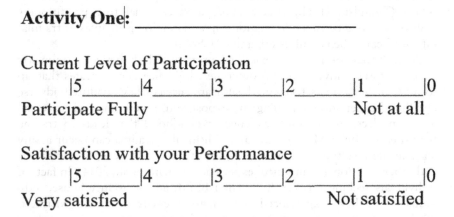

Figure 14.2 Activity Card Sort participation and satisfaction rating scale.
Source: Tyminski et al., 2020.

The results of John's evaluation indicate that, prior to homelessness and battling addiction, he had an increased level of participation in many education, social, leisure, and instrumental activities of daily living. The inclusion of the dark side of occupation into the assessment provides a better picture of the impact that homelessness and substance abuse have on John's occupational participation. John reported currently spending a large amount of his time in occupations related to finding and using substances, resource seeking, and other occupations necessary for survival (e.g. protecting my things, getting money, dealing with stress and emotions). When looking ahead to treatment planning for John, the occupational therapy practitioner can explore how his participation in the dark side of occupation impacts his ability to increase independence. For example, it may be impractical to address money management with John while he is currently using substances, or his participation in a typical workday due to shelters' restrictions on entry and exit times.

The use of the ACS-AIP allows the practitioner to explore the changes in participation as a result of experiencing homelessness or addiction. This information can be vital in intervention planning and goal setting. Further, understanding the impact that participation in the dark side of occupation has on overall engagement provides a more holistic view of the individual, thus creating opportunities for practitioners to address these occupations during intervention.

The importance of trauma-informed care

When addressed during the pilot study of feasibility for the ACS-AIP, most participants reported feeling slightly uncomfortable with discussions regarding sex, substance use, and relationships with family and significant others (Tyminski et al., 2020). Thus, it is essential that practitioners develop a strong therapeutic relationship and employ principles of trauma-informed care when administering the ACS-AIP.

A multitude of research exists to provide a link between traumatic experiences and adverse health outcomes. Evidence demonstrates that up to 30% of individuals receiving healthcare services have endured adverse childhood experiences, meaning any exposure to severe physical or sexual abuse, neglect, or domestic violence in childhood that leads to trauma (Felitti et al., 1998; Muskett, 2013). Additionally, trauma can occur at any stage in life resulting from an experience of violence, abuse, loss, disaster, and other emotionally impactful experiences (Huang et al., 2014). In fact, of individuals seeking services for mental health and substance abuse, individuals who have experienced trauma are the largest subset (Muskett, 2013). Practitioners must employ trauma-informed care to provide sensitive healthcare services for persons who have experienced trauma.

Trauma-informed care helps practitioners understand the impact trauma may have on an individual, recognise the signs and symptoms of trauma, and incorporate trauma-informed practices to prevent re-traumatisation (Substance Abuse and Mental Health Services Administration (SAMHSA), 2014). Trauma-informed care is practised at the programme, organisation, or system level. There are six key principles of trauma-informed care: safety, trustworthiness and transparency, peer support, collaboration and mutuality, empowerment, and cultural and gender issues (see Table 14.2).

Table 14.2 Six key principles of trauma-informed care

Safety	Individuals must feel physically and psychologically safe in their environment and interactions
Trustworthiness and Transparency	Individuals or organisations must gain the trust of the persons they serve
Peer Support	Promote support and sharing among individuals with the lived experience of trauma
Collaboration and Mutuality	All staff should be trained in trauma awareness and model the importance of positive relationships that promote recovery
Empowerment	Individuals and organisations implement a strength-based approach to treatment and look to clients for input on every aspect of treatment
Cultural and Gender Issues	Limit biases and provide care that is sensitive and inclusive of many cultures

Source: Hopper, Bassuk, & Olivet, 2010; SAMHSA, 2014.

Concluding recommendations

Based on the principles of trauma-informed care, administration of the ACS-AIP should occur in a location where the client reports feeling physically and psychologically safe. The occupational therapy practitioner providing the assessment should utilise principles of therapeutic use of self to create a therapeutic relationship that is sensitive to cultural and gender continuum needs, provides the client with a voice, and promotes trauma awareness (Solman & Clouston, 2016). Finally when reviewing the results of the assessment, it may be imperative to utilise a strength-based approach, concentrating on the assets a client possesses; thus, to focus on participation in health-giving occupations, while acknowledging the impact the participation in the dark side of occupation can have on the entire picture of the client's occupational identity.

References

Aldrich, R.M., Rudman, D.L., & Dickie, V.A. (2017). Resource seeking as occupation: A critical and empirical exploration. *American Journal of Occupational Therapy, 71*(3). doi:10.5014/ajot.2017.021782.

Baum, C.M. (2019). Secondary card sort. Unpublished research data. St. Louis, MO. Washington University School of Medicine.

Baum, C.M., & Edwards, D.F. (2008). *Activity Card Sort (ACS): Test manual* (2nd ed.). Bethesda, MD: AOTA Press.

Clark, F., Parham, D., Carlson, M.E., Frank, G., Jackson, J., Pierce, D., Wolfe, R.J., & Zemke, R. (1991). Occupational science: Academic innovation in the service of occupational therapy's future. *American Journal of Occupational Therapy, 45*(4), pp. 300–310. https://doi.org/10.5014/ajot.45.4.300.

Felitti, V., Anda, R., Nordenberg, D., Williamson, D., Spitz, A., Edwards, V., Koss, M., & Marks, J. (1998). Relationship of childhood abuse and household dysfunction to many of the leading causes of death in adults: The Adverse Childhood Experiences (ACE) study. *American Journal of Preventative Medicine, 14*(4), pp. 245–258. https://doi.org/10.1016/S0749-3797(98)00017-8.

Hopper, E.K., Bassuk, E.L., & Olivet, J. (2010). Shelter from the storm: Trauma-informed care in homeless services settings. *Open Health Services and Policy Journal, 3*, 80–100, doi:10.2174/1874924001003010080.

Huang, L.N., Flatow, R., Biggs, T., Afayee, S., Smith, K., Clark, T., & Blake, M. (2014). *SAMHSA's concept of trauma and guidance for a trauma informed approach* (SMA No. 14-4884). Retrieved from U.S. Department of Health and Human Services, Substance Abuse and Mental Health Services Administration. http://store.samhsa.gov/shin/content/SMA14-4884/SMA14-4884.pdf.

Kinebanian, A., & Stomph, M. (2010). Diversity matters: Guiding principles on diversity and culture. *World Federation of Occupational Therapists Bulletin, 61*, pp. 5–13. doi:10.1179/otb.2010.61.1.002.

Law, M., Baptiste, S., McColl, M., Opzoomer, A., Polatajko, H., & Pollock, N. (1990). The Canadian Occupational Performance Measure for occupational therapy. *Canadian Journal of Occupational Therapy, 57*(2), pp. 82–87. doi:10.1177/000841749005700207.

Muskett, C. (2013). Trauma-informed care in inpatient mental health settings: A review of the literature. *International Journal of Mental Health Nursing*, 23(1), pp. 51–59. doi:10.1111/inm.12012.

Rogers, E. (1995). *Diffusion of innovations* (4th ed.). New York: Free Press.

Rogers, E. (2002). Diffusion of preventative innovations. *Addictive Behaviors*, 27(6), pp. 989–993. doi:10.1016/S0306-4603(02)00300-3.

Rubio, D.M., Schoenbaum, E.E., Lee, L.S., Schteingart, D.E., Marantz, P.R., Anderson, K.E., … Esposito, K. (2010). Defining translational research: Implications for training. *Academic Medicine: Journal of the Association of American Medical Colleges*, 85(3), pp. 470–475. doi:10.1097/ACM.0b013e3181ccd618.

Sainburg, R.L., Liew, S.L., Frey, S.H., & Clark, F. (2017). Promoting translational research among movement science, occupational science, and occupational therapy. *Journal of Motor Behavior*, 49(1), pp. 1–7. doi:10.1080/00222895.2016.1271299.

Solman, B., & Clouston, T. (2016). Occupational therapy and therapeutic use of self. *British Journal of Occupational Therapy*, 79(8), pp. 514–516. doi:10.1177/0308022616638675.

Substance Abuse and Mental Health Services Administration (2014). SAMHSA's concept of trauma and guidance for a trauma-informed approach. Rockville, MD: Substance Abuse and Mental Health Service Administration.

Titler, M.G. (2018). Translation research in practice: An introduction. *OJIN: The Online Journal of Issues in Nursing*, 23(2), Manuscript 1. doi:10.3912/OJIN. Vol.23No02Man01.

Townsend, E., & Wilcock, A.A. (2004). Occupational justice and client-centered practice: A dialogue in process. *Canadian Journal of Occupational Therapy*, 71(2), pp. 75–87. doi:10.1177/000841740407100203.

Twinley, R. (2013). The dark side of occupation: A concept for consideration. *Australian Occupational Therapy Journal*, 60(4), pp. 301–303. doi:10.1111/1440-1630. 12026.

Twinley, R. (2017). The dark side of occupation. In K. Jacobs & N. MacRae (Eds.), *Occupational therapy essentials for clinical competence* (3rd ed., pp. 29–36). Thorofare, NJ: Slack.

Tyminski, Q. P., Drummond, R.R., Heisey, C., Evans, S., Hendrix, R., Jaegers, L.A. & Baum, C.M. (2020). Initial development of the Activity Card Sort- Advancing Inclusive Participation from a Homeless Population Perspective. *Occupational Therapy International*. https://doi.org/10.1155/2020/9083082.

Westfall, J.M., Mold J., & Fagnan L. (2007). Practice-based research – "Blue Highways" on the NIH roadmap. *Journal of the American Medical Association*, 297(4), pp. 403–406. doi:10.1001/jama.297.4.403.

Yerxa, E.J., Clark, F., Frank, G., Jackson, J., Parham, D., Pierce, D., Stein, C., & Zemke, R. (1989). An introduction to occupational science: A foundation of occupational therapy for the 21st century. *Occupational Therapy in Health Care*, 6(4), pp. 1–17.

Part IV

Occupational therapy education

15 Occupational therapy sounds too nice

Reflections from a recently trained occupational therapist

Kwaku Agyemang

Being a student

The very first essay I had to write as an occupational therapy student was to describe, explain and discuss how occupational therapists may use a range of the profession's core skills to support clients' health and wellbeing. This was an interesting piece of work as it focused my attention on all things occupational therapy and all the things we could do to assist individuals in attaining the most meaningful life possible for themselves. Through this, I discovered how complex the occupations we all as human beings choose or have to engage in really are.

As the first year of my training progressed, I began to question my understanding of meaningful occupations, as this was one of the main pillars of occupational therapy being taught to us. I started to question, what makes an occupation meaningful? Is this subjective? Does it have to be gender-specific to hold meaning? Does it have to be instrumental? Does it matter if it is not culturally specific? Can everyone describe their meaningful occupations? I struggled to answer, or to find answers, to all of these questions; what is more, I continued to lack any concrete understanding throughout the infancy of my training. That said, one core belief of the profession I grasped quickly was that health and wellbeing can be greatly affected by participation in occupations (Whalley Hammell & Iwama, 2012) and that satisfaction can be derived from doing so (Creek, 2002).

Early on during my second year at university I remember sitting in a lecture and thinking "Occupational therapy sounds too nice". I felt that most of what I was hearing and reading was directing me to work with an individual's diagnosis. In some way, this was understandable as a diagnosis can help with identifying symptoms; an understanding of symptoms, individually experienced, could then influence the degree to which an individual could engage in their occupations of choice, leading to a person-centred way of working. Throughout most of my studies, I recall there being a strong focus on health-promoting occupations individuals choose to engage in, such as exercise, cooking, and gardening, amongst many others. This also made sense to me, as some meanings, values, and beliefs individuals attached to these occupations meant that their health and wellbeing could be maintained through engagement in these occupations. On the other hand, it felt to me that there was not much emphasis placed on the values and beliefs that some individuals may have attached to other occupations; I thought about occupations which may be deemed to be unacceptable or health-compromising by the society in which an individual lives, such as substance use or those occupations associated with the use of violence. As I write this, I can see that my thoughts should not surprising, especially as, traditionally, occupational therapy philosophy has reinforced many assumptions regarding occupation, such as its positive contributions to health; there has certainly been a limited consideration of less positive, meaningful, or healthy experiences of occupations (Whalley Hammell, 2009).

Following this particular lecture, I spoke to a fellow student about my thoughts and she reflected that she shared this feeling. At this juncture, I felt I had a good understanding of the impact socially acceptable occupations could and do have on health and wellbeing. I was also beginning to understand how occupational therapists could use their activity or occupational analysis skills to adapt occupations to bring about improvements in health and wellbeing. Nevertheless, I remained concerned; I was apprehensive about the potential that I – as a qualified occupational therapist – might consciously and unconsciously pass judgement on the occupations individuals I work with choose to engage in to maintain their own version of health and wellbeing.

Occupational therapists: what are they doing?

Despite my awareness of this, I often wondered if occupational therapists working in, for example, forensic units ever explored the occupations individuals in their care engaged in which may perhaps have caused them to be in the forensic setting in the first instance. Again, I had questions to answer: Are the occupational therapists in such services concentrating on the occupations which neatly fitted into the three domains of self-care, productivity, and leisure? Were the occupational therapists in these settings, rehabilitation wards especially, solely focusing on individuals finding new occupations without an exploration of meanings they attached to previous occupations? This inquisitiveness led me to research the role of occupational therapists in forensic settings further. I did not have access directly to occupational therapists working in these settings so I was limited to reading online and speaking to the occupational therapists who were supervising me at this time in my employed role in a mental health rehabilitation unit and also learning disability assessment and treatment service.

The dark side of occupations

Encountering the concept of the dark side of occupations changed the direction I wanted to go with my occupational therapy career. I recall a very cold and foggy Saturday morning in September 2016, when two fellow enthusiastic occupational therapy students and I made the journey to Duxford, Cambridgeshire for a study day about the dark side of occupations. This is where I met Dr Twinley and what I heard throughout the day really inspired me and challenged my thinking. Having been directed throughout my studies to always take an occupational perspective and remain occupation-focused in my work, this concept complemented my learning as it answered many of the questions I had had earlier in my studies. I felt an urge and eagerness to further understand why people were in forensic units and what types of occupations they choose or had chosen in the past to engage in. I wanted to look beyond the set domains of self-care, leisure, and productive occupations which people engaged in on a daily basis. Having the confidence as an occupational therapist to look beyond these set domains with the client, to me, felt I would be achieving a more client-centred practice. Collaboration being one of the core skills of practice, it is paramount that it is used during engagement with clients, especially when exploring occupations which have not traditionally been readily discussed. This skill can empower those we work with to share more about these occupations. It can also be reparative in terms of some of the experiences they have had in the past with those in authority or other professional services they have come across.

I am aware that the term the dark side of occupation has received some negative critique (Kiepek, Beagan, Rudman, & Phelan, 2019; Pettican, 2018). When I first became aware of the term, however, I did not personally attribute any negative inferences to it. Some have suggested the term could infer harmful racial overtones or attract negativity in terms of the links darkness has with unhappiness or unpleasantness. I can certainly understand and appreciate these concerns, especially if the individual with these concerns has been in a situation where the word "dark" has been used as a derogatory term towards them. In the context of occupation, however, to me, the term provides an opportunity to be aware of the occupations which may not be readily explored during initial contact with the people I work with. It allows me to come from a place of curiosity about the occupations people choose to engage in, and to do so regardless of my own opinions of them as being either positive or negative, acceptable or unacceptable, healthy or unhealthy, for instance.

Shaming, labelling, and assuming

Twinley's concept has also facilitated me to consider the impact of shaming, labelling, and making assumptions about the things other people do. When it comes to occupations that are deemed socially unacceptable, some people may feel a sense of shame about these occupations due to their awareness of society's perceptions of them. Yet, on the other hand, the meaning and purpose they gain from these occupations could counteract, or lessen, the shame they may experience at times. On the topic of what is deemed socially acceptable, I have become increasingly aware that occupations that challenge social norms were perhaps also not explored due to learnt assumptions on the part of the occupational therapist about them. From experience, I can recall scenarios where a general assumption must have been made by the occupational therapist and their client – even in situations where both were aware that some occupations the client experiences could be viewed as antisocial, there seems to have been a subconscious decision not to explore it. This is the responsibility of the occupational therapist; we must challenge assumptions and facilitate a more open exploration of people's occupational needs and potential. Occupational therapists are skilled in assessing and understanding the impact and also the power of occupation. We should therefore try not to let our own views on occupations detract from our ability to explore them. Following an initial contact with a client, especially if it was a particularly difficult contact, it is very easy for us all to be emotionally charged and therefore to label/make assumptions about the impact occupations were having on them. We, as occupational therapists, however, have to be able to control our emotional responses and remember to use our occupational lens to fully understand the meaning and value the client is placing on the occupation. It could be argued that making an assumption could lead some occupational therapists into carelessly labelling their clients' occupations as "dark". Twinley (2017) however asserts that her intention in using the term "the dark side of occupations" was to act as a prompt for occupational therapists to consider occupations which remain explored from an occupational perspective. This was also my understanding, rather than using it as a term to label other people's occupations.

Critical reflexivity

Learning about the concept of the dark side of occupation has led me to develop critical reflexivity in relation to my practice. During the very early stages of my training, my own assumptions about occupations and how and why people engaged in them were developed through no fault of those who taught me. The reasons why I had chosen to study occupational therapy were partly based on my idealistic views of the world. My personal beliefs somewhat matched some of the core beliefs of the profession, which caused me no concern at the inception of my studies. However, as I continue to learn more about myself and the world around me, I have developed a strength in identifying and unlearning some of the assumptions and views placed on the occupations people around me and clients I work with engage in. This critical reflexivity therefore allows me not to be fearful of exploring the occupations the clients I work with engage in, which are often ones the society in which I live considers not to be healthy, productive, or prosocial. I have learnt from clients that some of their occupations have not always been done out of choice, but instead out of necessity or coercion. With time, by engaging in critically reflexive practice I have developed the confidence to ask questions about less explored occupations; for me, this is about critically considering the impact of my assumptions, values, and even actions as I work with clients, and on the work that we do. To illustrate, during my third practice placement in a medium secure unit I recall undertaking an interview alongside my educator with an individual who had a history of engaging in violence and sexual deviance. As I had begun to gain an understanding of the purpose of the dark side of occupation concept, I really wanted and wished for my educator to ask about his engagement in violence, and to explore if he attributed any meaning to it. I was hoping I would be able to hear the types of questions which would be asked in order to explore this, but this did not occur. The more understanding I gained about the dark side of occupation through reading, the more evident it became that the line of questioning should not differ from those questions which would be asked of occupations mostly deemed as prosocial and health-promoting. Working as an occupational therapist in a prison setting with young offenders, and exploring their engagement in all occupations, it is evident that reasons behind their engagement are multifaceted. These reasons are also all subjective. There are, however, some commonalities experienced by the young people, such as the impact of having a poor or dysfunctional social environment, and also having a disrupted education. Education and attending school is one of the main occupations for the young people I work with. When this is disrupted by whatever means, the young people often report experiencing a compromised sense of wellbeing. This is often experienced as abandonment and rejection by the adults they felt could contain their emotions and provide them with a sense of safety. The combination of feelings and disrupted education could potentially leave the young people having a disregard of authority and lack of opportunities which, feasibly, can then be played out in them engaging in less desirable occupations.

My key learning points

- Something important I took from my placement in a medium secure unit was that there was a reason and meaning for everything people chose to do. Those reasons may not be very clear initially to the occupational therapist, but through exploration of people's engagement in any occupations it will, as I have found, become clearer.
- In my work with young offenders, I have had the opportunity to gain deeper insights into the values and beliefs individuals hold when it

comes to their engagement in occupations which may be considered as socially unacceptable, illegal, unhealthy, damaging, and disruptive. Gaining some insight into their subjective experiences has, I feel, provided me with a more comprehensive understanding which, in turn, helps me to plan more genuine and effective interventions.

- An individual should never label another person's occupations as "dark", regardless of personal views or opinions about the occupation.
- Using some of our core skills, such as therapeutic use of self and collaboration, can be really helpful when seeking to explore occupations that have previously remained unexplored.

My final thoughts

Reflecting on the formation of the profession, Creek (2002) suggests one of the founding beliefs is that humans could have an effect on their own health and wellbeing by being adept in occupations which allow exploration and interaction with the environment they are in. Thinking about the impact of environments, an individual living in a difficult and chaotic environment may engage in occupations instrumentally as a means for survival. I offer my final thoughts here based on my work experience: I have come to appreciate the diverse reasons economically deprived people, for instance, may choose to engage in shoplifting for food. Within the social context of welfare cuts and an increased need for food banks, it is hypothesised that survival is the main driver for engaging in shoplifting (Strachan, 2018). Beyond this, aside from fulfilling their need for food and lessening their hunger, risk, excitement, and improving the skills required to successfully shoplift can be equally important reasons and motivational factors. As a second example, it is known that children born into and living in households where family members have a history of substance use disorder are at an increased likelihood to also use substances (Lipari & Van Horn, 2017). Growing up in a household where drug taking is commonplace and normalised may well sustain an individual's engagement with this occupation, regardless of its impact upon the state of their health and wellbeing. Besides addiction, sustained engagement in this occupation may also be due to an individual's desire to meet other needs, such as providing opportunities to form what they perceive or experience to be meaningful relationships with family members – thus, attaching a strong value to this occupation.

As a recently qualified occupational therapist, I think consideration should be given to this concept, its meanings and intentions, especially by academics working in occupational therapy departments; you are responsible for training budding occupational therapy students who need to be encouraged to learn about and apply occupation and occupational science concepts early on in their studies. Just as I have found, the confidence to explore the previously unexplored can be boosted with the understanding that not all occupations people engage in are addressed in practice; this includes those that are not legal, productive, or health-promoting, but that still hold meaning and value to an individual. This is not to promote further engagement in that particular occupation, nor to advocate for it, but to gain insight as to what is really meaningful to a person, and whether similar values could be derived from other occupations.

References

Creek, J. (Ed.) (2002). *Occupational therapy and mental health.* London: Churchill Livingstone.

Kiepek, N.C., Beagan, B., Rudman, D.L., & Phelan, S. (2019). Silences around occupations framed as unhealthy, illegal, and deviant, *Journal of Occupational Science, 26*(3), pp. 341–353. doi:10.1080/14427591.2018.1499123.

Lipari, R.N., & Van Horn, S.L. (2017). Children living with parents who have a substance use disorder. The CBHSQ Report. Retrieved from www.samhsa.gov/data/sites/default/files/report_3223/ShortReport-3223.html.

Pettican, A. (2018). "Getting together to play football" A participatory action research study with the Positive Mental Attitude Sports Academy (Doctoral dissertation, University of Essex, UK). Retrieved from http://repository.essex.ac.uk/24364/1/1%20Master%20and%20appendicies%20doc.pdf.

Strachan, G. (2018, 21 June). 'Survival' shoplifting rise linked to austerity. *The Courier.* Retrieved from www.thecourier.co.uk/fp/news/local/angus-mearns/674287/survival-shoplifting-rise-linked-to-austerity/.

Twinley, R. (2017). The dark side of occupation. In K. Jacobs & N. MacRae (Eds.), *Occupational therapy essentials for clinical competence* (3rd ed., pp. 29–36). Thorofare, NJ: Slack.

Whalley Hammell, K.R. (2009). Sacred texts: A sceptical exploration of the assumptions underpinning theories of occupation. *Canadian Journal of Occupational Therapy, 76*(1), pp. 6–13. https://doi.org/10.1177/000841740907600105.

Whalley Hammell, K.R., & Iwama, M.K. (2012). Well-being and occupational rights: An imperative for critical occupational therapy. *Scandinavian Journal of Occupational Therapy, 19*(5), pp. 385–394. doi:10.3109/11038128.2011.611821.

16 The dark side of studying at university

Priscilla Ennals

The occupation of studying at university

Participating in, and succeeding at, the occupation of studying at university, requires students to engage in sustained occupational effort: persisting with a series of activities over a number of years. Many of these relate directly to studying, for example, attending classes, completing assignments and exams, engaging in work placements or fieldwork in many courses, engaging in group work, reading prescribed texts, revising, and researching. Simultaneously students must engage in all the occupations that sustain their lives, for example, relationships with family and friends, self-care, maintaining or contributing to a home, employment, travel, relaxation, and leisure activities. Students living independently and financially supporting themselves typically have a wider range of demands than those supported by family and still living at home (Richardson, Elliott, Roberts, & Jansen, 2017). However, we also know that some students have caring roles and that family expectations about succeeding at study can be experienced as a heavy burden. Poverty and housing insecurity can also be challenges. Thinking about the experience of being a university or college student therefore requires a wide occupational lens that extends well beyond a sole focus on education.

Studying while living with mental ill health

My doctoral studies involved investigating the experiences of university students who were living with mental ill health (see Box 16.1 for a summary of the study). The central finding was that students felt both capable and different, and had to manage feeling different in order to persist with studying. The participating students revealed the occupations they engaged in and those that they avoided as a way of managing their sense of distress and difference. These covered a spectrum from occupations that could be described as positive and health-promoting, to those that would be described as negative, unhealthy, self-defeating, risky, or even life-threatening. When feeling most different or distressed, students described using strategies that were typically towards the negative end of the spectrum. For example, drinking alcohol before classes as a way of having the courage to get there and to participate in a chemistry lab or a tutorial; using laxatives, fasting or purging to maintain a sense of control; and cutting and burning one's own body to manage distress. Not doing activities required for success at study, e.g. not attending classes or doing the required work outside of class, also featured in their descriptions. Instead they engaged in alternative occupations, for example, gaming for many hours a day, watching social media passively or participating in the dark web (websites on an encrypted network that cannot be accessed using traditional search engines), drinking or using drugs, or sleeping through days; all facilitating avoidance of activities they knew they needed to be doing. See Box 16.2 for an example of one participant's occupational strategies. Often these were described not as active choices or as occupations that were desirable; but they were purposeful, as strategies for avoiding or managing the distress associated with living, with negotiating early adulthood, and with striving to be a university student – an occupation they each found highly meaningful and desirable, and one they were committed to succeeding at.

Box 16.1 A grounded theory study of the experiences of university students living with mental ill health (Ennals, 2016)

My doctoral study sought to better understand the experience of studying at university for students living with mental ill health. I used constructivist grounded theory (Charmaz, 2014) and a participatory framework where the intention was to research *with* people rather than conduct research on people (Reason & Bradbury, 2008). It was conducted at one Australian University. The central participatory mechanism was a reference group overseeing the study, that involved people with lived experience of mental ill health and studying at university. Data were gathered through 21 in-depth interviews with 15 students and 12 recorded reference group meetings. The students were aged 21 to 39 years old, two-thirds were female, and two-thirds were undertaking bachelor's degrees. Most had diagnoses of depression or anxiety. Psychosis, bipolar disorder and post-traumatic stress disorder were each experienced by two participants.

The study found that students who participated were striving to be 'regular' university students and felt both capable and different in their efforts to be students. They had to find ways to manage the sense of difference they experienced, using different strategies depending on the degree of difference they felt at any time. When the demands of studying outweighed their resources, they dropped out of study, however all had found ways to return to study when I interviewed them. The study identified the forces that confirm difference, including silencing, isolation and categorising, and the processes that open space for difference, including speaking out, connecting and successful doing.

Box 16.2 "Brad's" experience

Brad was a 27-year-old first year student enrolled for the fifth time in a post-secondary course. He had not completed any of the previous courses. He had failed year 12 on his first attempt but succeeded the following year. He described a difficult childhood with his father dying by suicide when he was 8 years old. He struggled to make friends and felt alienated, turning to drinking and gaming in early adolescence. He described a long history of depression, with multiple efforts at intervention. He was receiving counselling and was registered with the university disability support service.

Brad described the despair he felt after dropping out of study on one occasion, first feeling "numb", then having a "hollow feeling", depression, apathy, hopelessness and thoughts of suicide. He described how he avoided the reality of his despair by "getting out of my head" through obsessive video gaming:

> I started a World of Warcraft addiction…. It is an escapism … because I started to feel depression, so computer games have been my escape for years. They let me cope by not thinking…. You stop studying, you spend more time playing games because if you're going to feel hollow you might as well just play games and not feel hollow.
>
> ("Brad")

His social life went from small to non-existent, where he left the house only to get food and did not speak to anyone. He took to bed and gaming, describing more than 16 hours of play a day, interspersed only by sleep. He sought help from the counselling service after hitting rock bottom and feeling like he couldn't fail again. He shared how suicidal thoughts had become a motivator. He was hopeful that he would make some friends and succeed at study.

Students also described the physical and social environmental contexts they occupied and how they managed levels of environmental demand and stimulation by seeking out or avoiding particular environments. These included effortful management to avoid or minimise social contact while on campus, blocking out noise and social contact by using headphones or focusing on their phones, seeking out quiet green spaces, quiet corners of buildings or the library, staying at home, or travelling during off-peak times. Similar strategies have been described in a range of other qualitative studies (Ennals, Fossey, & Howie, 2015).

While the participant cohort I was studying had all experienced mental ill health, describing formal diagnoses of schizophrenia, bipolar disorder, anxiety and depression, alongside many other experiences including trauma, abuse, poverty, or growing up in families with mental illness, I started thinking about university students more generally. In particular, the occupational therapy students that I came to know in my lecturer role. I started to wonder if these ways of managing distress were perhaps more prevalent and more universal than I had considered. I started to listen to their experiences differently and suspended my judgement about their motivations, choices, and the activities they were doing or not doing. I also reflected differently on my own time at university, both past and current as a doctoral candidate, and the strategies I had used, and was using; strategies that might be considered to span a wide spectrum of the scale from health-promoting to unhealthy, positive to negative. From my standpoint as occupational therapist, occupational scientist, lecturer, and student, I revised my thinking about *studying* as an occupation.

Studying: a complex occupation warranting further investigation

Studying is a complex, multifaceted occupation that frequently has a dark or shadow side for many students. With increasing rates of upper secondary education completions in many countries (OECD, 2018), post-secondary study is often positioned as the next developmental step. While it is seen as a positive occupation that increases career opportunities and future earning potential, it can also be experienced as demanding, stressful and a potential trigger for mental ill health. For students with additional challenges, including but not limited to mental ill health, the further challenge of managing difference can be an added burden. Yet this is rarely discussed by students or educators. The darker side of studying, and the "negative", "unhealthy", "maladaptive" actions taken to manage, may be a critical enabling factor in supporting many students, to sustain periods of peak demand such as exam periods, and the long haul of a university degree.

Being a university student and studying is desired by most who participated in the study I conducted. The students I spoke to perceived study as a means to a life and career they wanted, and a way of meeting their potential, of doing what they loved. They felt drawn to study, as a way of expanding their choices and life options. They were passionate about it, as something they were good at. They all felt capable as students and it was this sense of capacity that drew them to the role, even though several had dropped out of study or experienced multiple episodes of failure. See Box 16.3 which

Box 16.3 "Stacy's" experience

Stacy came reluctantly to Australia from Asia to study when she was 19, forced by her parents into a high-prestige course that was not her preferred choice. She knew she was a bright and capable student but found adapting to independent living and life away from her family difficult. Her strong family ties and cultural expectations meant that Stacy felt she had no choice but to persist with the course.

> Finally, one day, I just didn't want to touch my books anymore.... What I did was just have lots and lots of sleep. Then lots of crying sessions because I was scared. I couldn't perform, and exams were just around the corner.... I didn't want to live.

Since that first "breakdown" Stacy had twice dropped out of study and gone into hiding before eventually returning to her family. They brought her back to Australia to study after allowing some time to recuperate. At the time of her interview she had recently been supported by community mental health services after feeling acutely suicidal. When I shared during the interview that her experiences were common and that many other students also found studying and life difficult she expressed both astonishment and gratitude.

> I'm very encouraged by the fact that there's many people like me; not just me alone. I think that is what I need to hear, and that it is possible to overcome.

describes one participant, "Stacy's" experience of feeling capable but struggling in the student role.

Lessons about the dark side of studying

I came to wonder about the silence and shame that surround this darker side of occupational participation, and how when, as a profession, we emphasise the positive, health-promoting elements of participation we are party to this silencing and shaming; party to ignoring, denying or even suppressing major parts of many people's lives. I propose that shining a light on this darker side may facilitate different ways of thinking about the complexity of occupational participation, about what enables participation, and may support a more rounded and truly holistic view of occupation.

My study found that silencing was a mechanism for confirming difference. Not coping with studying, not coping with life as a university student, and the use of "negative" strategies for coping are rarely discussed and certainly not considered as acceptable – within the academic community or between students. If discussed, they are deemed as "problems" or "issues" to be addressed and resolved. For example, drug and alcohol use by students, or self-harming, or suicidal ideation are described with fear, positioned as things to be avoided, managed, and eliminated. This has been exacerbated through dominant biomedical conceptualisations of mental illness and distress, with messages of professional help-seeking assumed to be the only legitimate approach to supporting students (Jorm, 2012; Simpson & Ferguson, 2012). The stance of many universities currently is to identify and manage student mental ill health. When they cannot be managed, students are often managed out of the system. Students frequently manage this themselves by withdrawing from subjects or courses, or just drifting away from study, with mental ill health acknowledged as a contributor to high rates of course non-completion (Orygen – The National Centre of Excellence in Youth Mental Health, 2017).

Many students do not have peers to share their experiences with, and do not hear from others about similar struggles. For example, Stacy (Box 16.3) shared her belief that she was the only student in her cohort of 400 students who was struggling, who had failed, and was stunned to hear me refute this. My study found that when students had the opportunity to share their experiences, to hear the similar experiences of others, and to connect around these, they felt less alone in their struggle and despair, and more able to persist with study, despite feeling different. This strategy of connection, and raising awareness of the common struggle of many students, varies from an emphasis on identification of mental illness, help-seeking, and individualised treatment – the strategy currently favoured by universities. However, student-led organisations internationally are pushing back and taking up this challenge themselves, for example Batyr in Australia, the Mental Health Task Team in Stellenbosch, South Africa, Student Minds in the UK, and Active Minds in North America, are finding ways for students to share and hear stories of struggle and strength, to connect around their self-perceived difference and distress, and to feel less alone and less different as a result.

This affirms the need for our occupational theories to acknowledge and accommodate the dark side of occupation. To consider that many people experience some form of struggle in participating in occupations that matter to them. That many people use strategies that can be considered negative, unhealthy, or maladaptive to engage in occupations that hold personal value and meaning. That the routine effort of living and participating is frequently hard, involves both the light and dark, the positive, negative and everything in between – all of which can be acknowledged and accommodated within our overall intention towards wellbeing, health, and quality of life. The dark side should not only be considered as a problem and something to be managed or eliminated, but as part of a routine life.

Concluding thoughts

Is there a role for educators to play? If we create opportunities for discussing the potential for struggle and challenge in student life, and in the occupation of studying, those students who are feeling different, alone, or distressed may recognise the shared nature of their experience, and the enabling nature of the strategies they use to sustain their participation. Instead of positioning these activities as harmful, maladaptive, or negative they can be seen through this expanded occupational lens as occupationally adaptive (Frank, 1996; Nayar & Stanley, 2015). They may also come to see that there are myriad ways of dealing with difficult experiences apart from concealing their distress, withdrawing, or numbing through substance use, self-harming, bingeing, purging, or obsessive gaming. It may raise awareness that strategies such as speaking out, connecting with others, seeking help, and accepting difference can ease the passage (Laidlaw, McLellan, & Ozakinci, 2015), and may enhance their study experience.

References

Charmaz, K. (2014). *Constructing grounded theory* (2nd ed.). Thousand Oaks, CA: Sage.

Ennals, P. (2016). Capable and different: A grounded theory of studying at university for students experiencing mental ill-health (Doctoral dissertation, La Trobe University, Melbourne, Australia). Retrieved from http://arrow.latrobe.edu.au:8080/vital/access/manager/Repository/latrobe:41915?queryType=vitalDismax&query=ennals.

Ennals, P., Fossey, E., & Howie, L. (2015). Postsecondary study and mental ill-health: A meta-synthesis of qualitative research exploring students' lived experiences. *Journal of Mental Health, 24*(2), pp. 111–119. doi:10.3109/09638237.2015.1019052.

Frank, G. (1996). The concept of adaptation as a foundation for occupational science research. In R. Zemke & F. Clark (Eds.), *Occupational science: The evolving discipline* (pp. 47–55). Philadelphia: F.A. Davis Company.

Jorm, A. (2012). Mental health literacy: Empowering the community to take action for better mental health. *American Psychologist, 67*(3), pp. 231–243.

Laidlaw, A., McLellan, J., & Ozakinci, G. (2015). Understanding undergraduate student perceptions of mental health, mental well-being and help-seeking behaviour. *Studies in Higher Education, 41*(12), pp. 2156–2168. doi:10.1080/03075079.2015.1026890.

Nayar, S., & Stanley, M. (2015). Occupational adaptation as a social process in everyday life. *Journal of Occupational Science, 22*(1), pp. 26–38. doi:10.1080/14427591.2014.882251.

OECD (2018). Education at a glance. Organization for Economic Development. Retrieved from www.oecd.org/education/education-at-a-glance.

Orygen – The National Centre of Excellence in Youth Mental Health (2017). Under the radar. The mental health of Australian university students. Retrieved from www.orygen.org.au/Policy/Policy-Reports/Under-the-radar/Orygen-Under_the_radar_report.

Reason, P., & Bradbury, H. (Eds.) (2008). *The SAGE handbook of action research: Participative inquiry and practice* (2nd ed.). London: Sage.

Richardson, T., Elliott, P., Roberts, R., & Jansen, M. (2017). A longitudinal study of financial difficulties and mental health in a national sample of British undergraduate students. *Community Mental Health Journal, 53*(3), pp. 344–352.

Simpson, A., & Ferguson, K. (2012). Mental health and higher education counselling services – responding to shifting student needs. *Journal of the Australian and New Zealand Student Services Association, 39*, pp. 1–12.

17 How the dark side of occupation can be instructed in a course

Learning from occupational therapy

Julie Nastasi

Context

The World Federation of Occupational Therapists (WFOT) provides approval/accreditation for occupational therapy education programs throughout the world. I work in the United States of America (USA), where occupational therapy education programs receive accreditation through the Accreditation Council for Occupational Therapy Education (ACOTE). *The Minimum Standards for the Education of Occupational Therapists* (WFOT, 2016) and *2018 Accreditation Council for Occupational Therapy Education (ACOTE®) Standards and Interpretive Guide* (ACOTE, 2018) provide occupational therapy educators throughout the world and in the USA, respectively, with the minimum requirements needed to develop and run an occupational therapy education program. Twinley's concept of the dark side of occupation is not specifically named in either accreditation document; this could be reflective of the fact that occupations such as those that are "uncomfortable" (e.g. sex), or those that involve high levels of risk, are harmful, or illegal, are more difficult to study, and so there is limited research to inform teaching and, therefore, curriculum development.

Encouragingly, occupational therapists and occupational scientists have started to respond to the call for occupations previously unexplored (or under-explored) to be studied and exposed; the very fact you are reading this text is indicative of this international response amongst our colleagues. The omittance of the dark side of occupation in accreditation documents does not exclude addressing these occupations in occupational therapy education programs, as both documents address minimum standards. Incorporating the dark side of occupation into broader areas of occupational analysis will allow students to understand and appreciate the importance of gaining a holistic perspective of their clients in order to better evaluate and provide client-centred interventions.

Incorporating the dark side of occupation into curriculum

Occupation is the core of occupational therapy and occupational science. Considering the dark side of occupation is about exploring occupations that may not support health and/or well-being (Twinley, 2013) this, therefore, requires an appreciation of the point that not all occupations promote or even sustain health and/or well-being. Students must be able to evaluate, analyse, and apply occupation (ACOTE, 2018). I propose that application and understanding of the interaction between person-occupation-environment are essential to facilitate this. Students need knowledge of how occupations contribute to health and how they negatively influence health (WFOT, 2016). Educators should incorporate the dark side of occupation into learning experiences as students gain knowledge in the areas of the person, occupation, and environment. Gaining knowledge of the dark side of occupation will provide students with a well-rounded view and approach to occupation, as they can learn about people's diverse subjective experience of, and engagement in, occupation.

Person

In order to first understand their clients, students must learn how to obtain a detailed occupational profile. An occupational profile provides information about the client's occupational history and experiences (American Occupational Therapy Association, 2014). Occupational therapy students need to develop skills in obtaining a detailed occupational profile of their clients. This includes identifying valued occupations and activities as well as daily, weekly, monthly, and seasonal patterns and routines. This can include occupations perceived as somewhat boring or mundane. However, in some settings, this will certainly mean students need to develop comfort in asking their clients questions about typically unexplored occupations like alcohol/drug use, crime, and those occupations that are sexually violent or exploitative (Twinley, 2017; Twinley & Morris, 2014; Twinley & Addidle, 2012). In order to build these skills, educators may use role-play or standardised clients as methods to provide students with experience (Baird & Baker, 2017; Bennett, Rodger, Fitzgerald, & Gibson, 2017). In the USA, some occupational therapy programs have hired individuals to portray the role of standardised clients to provide students with the opportunity to gain experience with clients they otherwise would not have access to in the learning environment. More commonly, occupational therapy programs use role-play to provide students with experience. Here, I demonstrate how this role-play can be directed:

- The educator assigns a student to take on the persona of the client. The educator needs to provide the learning objective, environment, and a

- case scenario to the student playing the client. The educator may develop a script, or provide the student with information about the dark side of occupation to address.
- After the role-play of the case scenario, an occupational profile is completed by all students.
- The educator should debrief the students and provide feedback (Baird & Baker, 2017). During the debriefing, the educator should facilitate conversation and reflection on the dark side of occupation that emerged during completion of the occupational profile.
- Afterwards, students observing the role-play scenario should offer feedback on observations made, both duirng the role-play and completion of the occupational profile.
- The educator can facilitate critical and reflective discussion, asking questions such as: What might they have done differently? What would they have wanted to learn more about? What are the ethical and moral issues this raises? What challenges and opportunities were presented?
- The educator should provide additional clarification or information based on the students' feedback. If the educator does not want to have a student take on the role of client, a standardised client may be hired to act as the client. See Table 17.1 for examples of case scenarios.

Table 17.1 Case scenarios

Client 1	Client 2
James is a 23-year-old male who sustained a traumatic brain injury from a motor vehicle accident. He works in a bar as a bartender and also as a male prostitute. James lives in a flat with two other roommates. He has a history of alcohol and drug abuse. His work as a prostitute is important to him.	XL is a 28-year-old male who sustained multiple gunshot wounds. He is a member of a street gang and works in a pawn shop. XL has a girlfriend and two small children. He lives with his girlfriend and financially supports her and their two children.

Client 3	Client 4
Jill is a 40-year-old female, married with three kids, who fell and broke her arm. She is a "stay-at-home mum". She enjoys working out with friends, shopping, and recreational use of drugs. Her husband is a CEO of a company and they live comfortably in a wealthy neighbourhood, outside of a large city.	Jane is a 25-year-old female with an eating disorder. She lives with her boyfriend and comes to occupational therapy with visible bruises on her extremities. She and her boyfriend live in a rural area five hours away from her family. Jane has a history of missing work and frequently changes jobs.

Occupation

The minimum standards for WFOT and ACOTE require occupational therapy programs to address occupation (ACOTE, 2018; WFOT, 2016). This includes cultural and environmental influences on occupation (WFOT, 2016). Students need to analyse, adapt, and grade occupations (ACOTE, 2018; WFOT, 2016). The dark side of occupation also needs to be analysed to gain a better understanding of what qualities or characteristics are being sought out and what, if any, other occupations might be potential substitutes or replacements for those occupations that do not promote health and well-being. Educators need to provide their students with the skills needed to break down the components of the dark side of occupation, and identify what makes those occupations purposeful and meaningful to the client. Are there other occupations that would be purposeful and meaningful that clients might choose to participate in that promote and/or sustain their health and/or well-being? Are the occupations being chosen because other family members and friends are engaging in them? As Nhunzvi and Galvaan's case study (Nicky) raises in Chapter 11, some occupational choices are made to survive or to feel a sense of belonging. Is the participation in a specific occupation forced? These are all considerations that students must think about and be able to discuss with their clients. For example, sexual intimacy is a regular part of adult life for most; however, human trafficking is not. A client who has been forced into human sexual trafficking is physically coerced, exposed to violence, rape, confinement, and subsequently experiences trauma (National Center for Injury Prevention and Control, 2019). Educators need to encourage occupational therapy students to see and understand that occupations that might be perceived positively by some can be experienced differently by others, and vice versa.

In addition, there are occupations where the risk of harm outweighs benefits of participation. To illustrate with an example of where person-occupation-environment interact, consider the world's air quality today and its impact upon our health when performing certain occupations. There are many cities across the globe where air quality is so poor that the danger to people's health outweighs the benefits of participating in exercise: "In cities such as Allahabad in India, or Zabol in Iran, the long-term damage from inhaling fine particulates could outweigh the usual health gains of cycling after just 30 minutes" (*Guardian*, 2019). Clients may not realise the damaging or harmful effects of certain occupations if they are marginalised and have not been exposed to healthy occupations. Educators need to prepare students to critically evaluate occupations that "challenge ubiquitous beliefs in a causal relationship between occupation and health" (Greber, 2013, p. 459). Understanding how and why clients participate in such occupations will see students and educators alike addressing the dark side of occupation.

Environment

The environment plays a role in supporting or hindering participation in occupations. It is important that educators train their students to evaluate the environment to identify how the environment supports health and well-being, and how the environment may influence engagement in the dark side of occupation. Students need to understand the relationship of the person-occupation-environment. The environment is influenced by societal needs, local health, legislation, and relevant local occupations (WFOT, 2016). Educators need to teach students to evaluate and analyse sociocultural, socio-economic, diversity factors, and determinants of health (ACOTE, 2018). Questions to pose include:

- How can you incorporate consideration of practice during and after a global pandemic, especially where the environment is an acutely inhibiting factor?
- Does the environment support engagement in [said] occupation?
- What are the crime rates, both locally and where they will practise?
- Is there regular public violence?
- Are clients afraid to go outside after the sun sets?
- Is it safe to travel alone?
- Have clients or their families been robbed, raped, or attacked?
- What is the home environment like?
- What is the work environment like?
- Are clients able to safely access shopping stores, work, and home?
- Do clients need to live where they live?
- Are there other options for living, work, and shopping?
- Is there safe affordable childcare available?

These are all questions that educators could have their students think about. Through role-play, educators can teach students to gain confidence in asking questions about the environment, and how the environment influences occupation. To achieve this, experiential learning (Knightbridge, 2014) and service trips (Keane & Provident, 2017) provide another mechanism to expose students to different environments. Occupational therapy educators should consider incorporating experiential learning and service trips into the curriculum to safely expose students to environments where they will be able to observe the dark side of occupation. Students need to gain experiences in different environments to see how the environment can support or hinder occupation. Where service trips are not an option, educators may select documentaries and news clips to show their students; this can bring the world to students in very real ways, as stories help us to understand. After viewing, educators can facilitate discussion on the dark side of occupation, based on the global stories in the documentaries and news clips. WFOT (2016) requires students to have knowledge and practice with a range of people in different contexts. ACOTE (2018) also requires students to demonstrate analysis of context and environments. Context includes cultural, personal, temporal, and virtual; while environments include the physical and social (AOTA, 2014). Contemporary occupational therapy education must prepare students to address the dark side of occupation in these contexts and environments.

Concluding recommendations

Occupational therapy education programs must meet minimum standards in order to obtain and maintain accreditation. The dark side of occupation is not specifically named by WFOT or ACOTE (WFOT, 2016; ACOTE, 2018). Both accreditation documents provide broad guidelines for the areas that need to be addressed in occupational therapy education programs. I have argued that a holistic approach to occupation requires educators, students, and therapists to address the dark side of occupation. Educators need to prepare students to evaluate and provide interventions for people who engage in occupations currently regarded as in the dark, or the shadows: the under-explored occupations. Accreditation documents are not prescriptive, and leave room for occupational therapy programs to align with the mission of the institution that they are housed in. Including the dark side of occupation throughout the occupational therapy curriculum will prepare students to meet the occupational needs of their clients and provide client-centred services.

References

Accreditation Council for Occupational Therapy Education (2018). *2018 Accreditation Council for Occupational Therapy Education (ACOTE) Standards and Interpretive Guide*. Bethesda: Accreditation Council for Occupational Therapy Education. Retrieved from www.aota.org/~/media/Corporate/Files/EducationCareers/Accredit/StandardsReview/2018-ACOTE-Standards-Interpretive-Guide.pdf.

American Occupational Therapy Association (AOTA) (2014). Occupational therapy practice framework: Domain and process (3rd ed.). *American Journal of Occupational Therapy*, 68(Suppl. 1), S1–S48. http://dx.doi.org/10.5014/ajot.2014.682006.

Baird, J., & Baker, N. (2017). Role-play. *OT Practice*, 22(7), pp. 18–21.

Bennett, S., Rodger, S., Fitzgerald, C., & Gibson, L. (2017). Simulation in occupational therapy curricula: A literature review. *Australian Occupational Therapy Journal*, 64(4), pp. 314–327. doi:10.1111/1440-1630.12372.

Greber, C. (2013). Re: the dark side of occupation: A concept for consideration. *Australian Occupational Therapy Journal*, 60(6), pp. 458–459.

Guardian (2019). Tipping point: revealing the cities where exercise does more harm than good. Retrieved from www.theguardian.com/cities/2017/feb/13/tipping-point-cities-exercise-more-harm-than-good.

Keane, E., & Provident, I. (2017). Combining online education with international service learning to increase cultural competence. *Internet Journal of Allied Health Sciences and Practice*, 15(3), Article 6.

Knightbridge, L. (2014). Experiential learning on an alternative practice placement: Student reflections on entry-level competency, personal growth, and future practice. *British Journal of Occupational Therapy*, 77(9), pp. 438–446. doi:10.4276/0308 02214X14098207540956.

National Center for Injury Prevention and Control (2019). Sex trafficking. Retrieved from www.cdc.gov/violenceprevention/sexualviolence/trafficking.html.

Twinley, R. (2013). The dark side of occupation: A concept for consideration. *Australian Occupational Therapy Journal*, 60(4), pp. 301–303. doi:10.1111/ 1440-1630.12026.

Twinley, R. (2017). Woman-to-woman rape and sexual assault, and its impact upon the occupation of work: Victim/survivors' life roles of worker or student as disruptive and preservative. *Work*, 56(4), pp. 505–517. doi:10.3233/Wor-172529.

Twinley, R., & Addidle, G. (2012). Considering violence: The dark side of occupation. *British Journal of Occupational Therapy*, 75(4), pp. 202–204. doi:10.4276/0308 02212X13336366278257.

Twinley, R., & Morris, K. (2014). Are we achieving occupation-focused practice? *British Journal of Occupational Therapy*, 77(6), p. 275. doi:10.4276/0308022 14X14018723137922.

World Federation of Occupational Therapists (2016). *Minimum Standards for the Education of Occupational Therapists*. London: World Federation of Occupational Therapists. Retrieved from www.wfot.org/assets/resources/COPYRIGHTED-World-Federation-of-Occupational-Therapists-Minimum-Standards-for-the-Education-of-Occupational-Therapists-2016a.pdf.

18 Not everything is rosy and not everyone wants to fix their garden

An Australian example of integrating the dark side of occupation into curriculum for final year students

Amelia Di Tommaso

Introduction

The World Federation of Occupational Therapists (WFOT) is the body responsible for ensuring consistent and cohesive occupational therapy practice and education internationally (WFOT, 2002). The WFOT's educational guidelines stipulate that occupation and its relationship to health and wellbeing are central concepts explored in university occupational therapy programmes (WFOT, 2008). Commonly, when referring to occupation and health within the profession, the connection is overwhelmingly positive. Even the World Federation of Occupational Therapists' definition of occupational therapy suggested that through the therapeutic use of occupation, occupational therapists can enable health and wellbeing for clients (WFOT, 2010). However, in 2010, Molineux described that engaging in occupation can have an impact, positive or negative, on health and wellbeing. Despite this, Twinley (2013, 2017) suggested that most occupational therapy literature, textbooks, and content presented to students does not adequately explore and examine those occupations deemed less positive or with health-reducing potential. Additionally, further under-explored is the meaning such occupations hold for people or clients of occupational therapy services. In response to such issues, the dark side of occupation was developed (Twinley, 2013).

Occupation and its therapeutic use in practice is occupational therapy's unique contribution to healthcare (Molineux, 2004; Reilly, 1962; Wilcock, 2000). Occupational therapists should utilise their knowledge of occupation to enable occupational performance and in turn impact the health and wellbeing of the people with whom they work (McLaughlin Gray, 1998). Occupation-centred practice ensures that the therapist places "occupation at the center of his or her professional reasoning and links everything he or she does to the core paradigm of occupational therapy" (Fisher & Bray-Jones, 2017, p. 241). However, little exploration and consideration have been given to those occupations which are not necessarily health-enhancing but still hold meaning for people. It is unclear from the literature whether occupational therapists can fulfil the central tenets of the profession and be occupation-centred in their practice if the full spectrum of occupations are not enabled or encouraged in professional therapeutic settings. The dark side of occupation may assist occupational therapy practitioners and theorists to provide clarity on this issue in the future.

Integrating the dark side of occupation into curriculum

To explore the issue of occupation-centred practice and the potentially overly positive representation of occupation in the profession, one university programme in Australia has integrated the dark side of occupation into their curriculum. In their fourth and final year, students of an undergraduate occupational therapy education programme complete a course which focuses on critically examining the underpinning philosophy and theories of occupational therapy, to ensure advanced knowledge and application for future practice. It is within this course that students examine the theory of the dark side of occupation. There are several reasons why the dark side of occupation concept was chosen, including to critique and examine theory that is emerging within the professional lexicon, to further critically examine occupation and occupation-centred practice and its application in the Australian practice context, and for students to increase their clinical reasoning in complex situations. Also, given the nature of the topic, it was thought that it would be a creative and engaging means for students to examine their occupational knowledge and application to date, and to develop a critical position on how they may use the dark side of occupation in their future practice.

Students were presented with a case study of a de-identified client with whom the lecturer had worked. The case study included experiences of working through the occupational therapy process with a client who was engaged in several health-compromising occupations which also formed the foundation of his social activities. The client wished to return to these occupations post-discharge. The case study provided a stimulus for discussion about how to get the balance between using the client's chosen occupations in therapy, educating the client and also hospital staff on the importance of occupations and their impact on health, but also ensuring that the restrictions of the practice context are taken into account. Additionally, various scenarios were presented that commonly occur in everyday occupational therapy practice in diverse settings, as well as more challenging occupation-centred practice examples where the students were required to discuss their ideas, questions, concerns, intervention proposals, and associated justifications to small groups or the entire cohort.

Methods for evaluation

Currently, there is no literature which illuminates the student experience of learning about the dark side of occupation. To evaluate whether the dark side of occupation was useful as a teaching tool and to uncover the students' perspectives, a qualitative study was designed for final year student occupational therapists who completed the Advanced Occupational Therapy course over a two-year period. Focus groups allow for collective conversations and can often be called a group interview (Kamberelis & Dimitriadis, 2013; Kitzinger, 1994). Focus group design allowed for discussion and uncovering of students' current perspectives of the dark side of occupation, in a non-threatening environment and allowed for free-flowing discussion. The "pedagogic function" behind focus groups is to develop collective engagement which enables dialogue to reach higher levels of understanding, critical reflection, and knowledge generation of a group's interests (Kamberelis & Dimitriadis, 2013, p. 546). Kitzinger (1994) stated focus group interviews purposefully use group interactions as part of the method of data collection. Focus groups can be valuable as a pre-research method as they help to prepare for future studies by providing information from wide-ranging discussion (Brown, 2015). Therefore, given the limited information about the topic and the sometimes-challenging nature of discussing the dark side of occupation, focus groups were conducted.

Students had to volunteer to participate in the focus groups, which were conducted after the course had been completed. The first focus group had eight students who participated. The following year's group had nine participants. The facilitator of the groups was not the teacher of the course, to mitigate any unequal power relationships and to ensure an open discussion. Students were asked questions about the positive and challenging aspects of learning about the dark side of occupation and how they may use the concept in their future practice. Each focus group ran for approximately 60–80 minutes in length. The focus groups were audio-recorded and transcribed verbatim. The transcripts formed the data set. Braun and Clarke's (2006) method of thematic analysis was employed to analyse the data and uncover themes about learning about the dark side of occupation. Transcripts were analysed separately, at different time intervals, to ensure that codes inductively emerged from the data. Once all coding was completed, the lists of codes from both transcripts were combined. Forming categories from the focus groups was completed and refined until themes were formed from the data set. Ethical clearance was received from the university's human research ethics committee.

Students' perspective of learning about the dark side of occupation

Overall, there was similarity in the findings across the two focus groups; this was not unexpected given students completed the same course, one year apart. In summary, the students felt they had highly developed knowledge of occupation but learning about the dark side of occupation allowed for a deeper understanding of theoretical knowledge. Considering that occupation could have benefits and limitations on health and wellbeing allowed the students to re-conceptualise how they thought about occupation. Consequently, students felt more prepared for their post-graduation practice. However, some students questioned whether the concept of the dark side of occupation would be able to be adequately explored in the workplace because of the lack of acceptance from other health professionals.

A deeper understanding of occupation

The first theme that emerged was that learning about the dark side of occupation created opportunities for creating and sharing deeper understandings of occupation and occupation-centred practice. Students in both focus groups already felt that their knowledge of occupation was highly developed due to being in the fourth year of a programme which has a significant focus on occupational science and contemporary occupational therapy philosophy and theory. However, studying the dark side of occupation enabled most students to be able to think more broadly and deeply about occupation. One student commented that learning about the dark side of occupation had not "changed my idea of occupation, more that it broadened my understanding of occupation and what we should be thinking about as professionals". Another student further detailed that although in the early years of the degree, occupation, and the positive and negative impact on health, is discussed, it is not the focus:

> I think we talk about the health benefits so much and it is mentioned once or twice in the first year that [occupation] is maybe not always so health promoting but that is not what we focus on, so you just don't really think of that occupation in that way, so it was nice to be reminded and extend this.

Similarly, "Kelly" acknowledged that although she knew occupation had an impact on health from the nature of occupation content in first year study, she:

Never gave it a second thought, I don't think that I really would have put this together and made sense of it if we didn't do it in class. I had too much going on in first year to really think deeply about this.

More often, however, students discussed that their experience of occupation in the curriculum was focused on health-positive connotations of occupation. With "Sarah" commenting:

From the beginning we were told and explored that occupation had a positive impact on health and then learning that sometimes occupation can have a negative impact on health, I was surprised, but looking at the other side of it I found really interesting and had never really thought about it before. So, it changed my idea of [occupation].

"Katie" also felt her knowledge of occupation had improved and changed, stating "I think it has just opened up this whole new world for me and it has become way more complex". Additionally, "James" stated "I feel like I have got a more well-rounded perspective on things now". This sentiment was common amongst the participants. Although students had a good understanding of occupation, they felt that learning about the dark side of occupation assisted to further develop their knowledge of occupation, particularly when focusing on occupations that may not be health-enhancing.

Feeling prepared for the future

Another theme that emerged was that by studying the dark side of occupation, students felt more prepared to practise as an occupational therapist in the future. Students detailed that as they were exposed to complex and challenging case studies, coupled with time to develop and consider their practice choices and justifications, this created a sense of confidence to graduate.

Feeling more prepared to practise as a new graduate occupational therapist was common amongst all students. "Anna" commented on being exposed to situations where clients may be interested in engaging in occupations that may not be commonly discussed in current practice settings or during classes at university, by stating:

I feel now I am so much better prepared to go out there and work in the real world because not everything is rosy and not everyone wants to fix their garden and make rice paper rolls and all that sort of stuff. So, it will make us better therapists for it.

"Melanie" also commented that she felt better prepared to justify her practice decisions if she was ever to enable a client to participate in occupations that may have a detrimental impact on health: "you know you can justify it, you can justify it to other professionals and then know that you'd be able to justify it if someone disagreed with that".

Students described that thinking differently about occupations that were not always health-enhancing but still had meaning to clients was particularly useful in developing their professional identity. Clare identified that by considering the dark side of occupation as a concept she may be more client-centred: "I think it is really going to have a positive effect on the relationship you have with your client too. For them to see that we are trying to understand things from their perspective." Finally, "Michelle" commented that learning about the dark side of occupation "helped me to really see the kind of therapist I could be".

Implementing the dark side of occupation in healthcare settings: a challenge

The perception that other health professionals would not be supportive of enabling all occupations and fully enacting the dark side of occupation concept to practice was consistent amongst all the participants. Sarah stated: "If you've made that decision to enable a person to engage in whatever [occupation], the biggest barrier to that is probably organisational staff or senior staff or your mentor saying, 'No, don't do that'". This sentiment clearly resonated with the students after reflecting on previous fieldwork experiences, as "Nicole" described:

> I think the influence of the people you're working with is the challenge; if you're working with other occupational therapists and they're like, "Oh, I'd never consider that, to enable them," I think it's going to be difficult to stray from the pack in that way as well.

Given the risk-averse, litigious nature of healthcare, students were hesitant about how the dark side of occupation could be implemented into practice. However, given the implications for occupation- and client-centred practice, some students felt they would continue to strive to apply this concept in their future practice. One student explained that being challenged in class and being given the opportunity to develop justifications and their clinical reasoning made them feel more prepared:

> I feel like it also gives you the language to justify your choices to other people in your team, to tell them why you are asking about more than you normally would be about clients' occupations, or why your intervention may look different. It is good to have something to underpin reasoning or what you're doing.

Therefore, implementing the dark side of occupation into university curriculum was beneficial to students to enable them to think more broadly about their practice, how their practice could be shaped by the perceptions of other health professionals, and to ensure that they feel prepared for their future practice.

Reflections on the teaching process

The findings from this small exploratory study highlighted that final year student occupational therapists benefited from learning about the dark side of occupation as it assisted them to deepen and evaluate their existing knowledge of occupation. Students universally felt that the dark side of occupation was "a much-needed topic to cover" and enhanced their feelings of preparedness for future practice. Insights from students about their experiences in the classroom have assisted to refine the delivery of emerging theory such as the dark side of occupation.

Developing authentic scenarios

During the development of the module and associated learning activities, as there were limited documented examples of how best to teach aspects of emerging theory and specifically the dark side of occupation, it was useful to draw on previous practice experiences; this also meant the curriculum was developed based on what students may realistically encounter in the future. Sharing anonymised case studies was beneficial for the students to see how using the theory of the dark side of occupation can be considered in practice. One student commented:

> I think it was helpful during class when the lecturer gave us examples of their experiences; that really helped me to get a solid example of when [the dark side of occupation] was practised in real life. So that really helped my understanding as well, getting a real-life example.

By using authentic practice scenarios, students were able to see how the confluence of personal values, clinical reasoning, theoretical and philosophical underpinnings of the profession, and consideration for the practice context combine for the best occupational outcome for a client.

Allowing for discussion to examine personal values and assumptions

Unsurprisingly, when students were discussing aspects of the dark side of occupation in class, their personal values and assumptions often came to the fore. At times it was challenging for some to reconcile their personal and professional values. Although students do examine their personal values and how these can impact on practice throughout their degree, it was beneficial to be reminded and to discuss this topic again. One student commented:

> I think just a reminder that we as therapists do have your own values and beliefs and that is always going to influence your practice, but that we actually have to be really mindful of how that influences our practice. This class was good to remember to be mindful of our own bias in practice.

Confronting bias and the impact that personal values have when implementing aspects of the dark side of occupation in practice was challenging for some students. However, some students felt these difficult discussions were beneficial as they could again reflect on the stereotypes they held about people who may engage in heath-limiting occupations. Interestingly, this also led to conversations about students' reflections of their own occupational participation and how they may engage in occupations that they may not see as enhancing health and wellbeing.

Creating a brave space in the classroom

Creating a safe space and ground rules in the classroom for respectful discussion is commonplace for all educators (Arao & Clemens, 2013). However, Arao & Clemens (2013) argued that there are limitations to creating safe spaces, including that the educator directs the discussion, and that marginalised voices or people from diverse cultural groups are not heard or do not feel comfortable to share. Therefore, educators have been challenged to create 'brave spaces' where discomfort with a topic should be acknowledged and the dominant discourse is questioned (Arao & Clemens, 2013; Verduzco-Baker, 2018). When designing curriculum to include the dark side of occupation, occupational therapy educators should reflect on how they can create brave spaces in the classroom to enable a respectful, yet in-depth discussion about how this theory could be implemented within the profession. Upon reflection, this topic required the students to feel comfortable with each other and to share diverse opinions. This content was well timed in the students' fourth and final year as a cohort, as they were familiar with each other and accustomed to sharing their opinions and clinical justifications without judgement. Students in the focus groups commented that they felt respected by their peers to share their opinions and rationale, even if their perspectives differed. Despite this, it was helpful to have focused stimulus questions to get the students to think about the dark side of occupation, and then to develop how they may use the concept within the occupational therapy process to ensure they were focused on the tasks and to meet the learning outcomes for the session.

Conclusion

All student occupational therapists must learn about the philosophical foundations of the profession to understand occupation and humans as occupational beings. However, the dominant narrative in education is that occupation enhances health and wellbeing. Learning about the dark side of occupation gave students a more in-depth and well-rounded perspective of occupation and provided an opportunity to refine their professional identity. Further research is required into how best to integrate the dark side of occupation into educational programmes internationally, and the impact this has on students' understanding of the central concepts of the profession.

References

Arao, B., & Clemens, K. (2013). From safe spaces to brave spaces: A new way to frame dialogue around diversity and social justice. In L.M. Landreman (Ed.), *The art of effective facilitation* (pp. 135–150). Sterling, VA: Stylus Publishing.

Braun, V., & Clarke, V. (2006). Using thematic analysis in psychology. *Qualitative Research in Psychology, 3*(2), pp. 77–101. doi:10.1191/1478088706qp063oa.

Brown, S. (2015). Using focus groups in naturally occurring settings. *Qualitative Research Journal, 15*(1), pp. 86–97. doi:10.1108/qrj-11-2013-0068.

Fisher, A., & Bray-Jones, K. (2017). Occupational therapy intervention process model. In J. Hinojosa, P. Kramer, & C. Royeen (Eds.), *Perspectives on human occupation: Theories underlying practice* (2nd ed., pp. 237–286). Philadelphia: F.A. Davis

Kamberelis, G., & Dimitriadis, G. (2013). *Focus groups: From structured interviews to collective conversations*. New York: Taylor & Francis.

Kitzinger, J. (1994). The methodology of focus groups: The importance of interaction between research participants. *Sociology of Health and Illness, 16*(1), pp. 103–121. doi:10.1111/1467-9566:ep11347023.

McLaughlin Gray, J. (1998). Putting occupation into practice: Occupation as ends, occupation as means. *The American Journal of Occupational Therapy, 52*(5), pp. 354–364. doi:10.5014/ajot.52.5.354.

Molineux, M. (2004). Occupation in occupational therapy: A labour in vain? In M. Molineux (Ed.), *Occupation for occupational therapists* (pp. 1–13). Oxford: Blackwell Publishing.

Molineux, M. (2010). The nature of occupation. In M. Curtin, M. Molineux, & J. Supyk-Mellson (Eds.), *Occupational therapy and physical dysfunction: Enabling occupation* (6th ed.). Edinburgh: Churchill Livingstone Elsevier.

Reilly, M. (1962). Occupational therapy can be one of the great ideas of 20th century medicine. *American Journal of Occupational Therapy, 16*(6), pp. 1–9.

Twinley, R. (2013). The dark side of occupation: A concept for consideration. *Australian Occupational Therapy Journal, 60*(4), pp. 301–303. doi:10.1111/1440-1630.12026.

Twinley, R. (2017). The dark side of occupation. In K. Jacobs & N. MacRae (Eds.), *Occupational therapy essentials for clinical competence* (3rd ed. pp. 29–36). Thorofare, NJ: Slack.

Verduzco-Baker, L. (2018). Modified brave spaces: Calling in brave instructors. *Sociology of Race and Ethnicity*, 4(4), pp. 585–592. doi:10.1177/2332649218763696.

Wilcock, A. (2000). Development of a personal, professional and educational occupational philosophy: An Australian perspective. *Occupational Therapy International*, 7(2), pp. 79–86. doi:10.1002/oti.108.

World Federation of Occupational Therapists (2002). *Revised minimum standards for the education of occupational therapists*. Perth: World Federation of Occupational Therapists.

World Federation of Occupational Therapists (2008). Position statement: Occupational Therapy entry-level qualifications. Retrieved from www.wfot.org/Resource Centre.aspx.

World Federation of Occupational Therapists (2010). Definitions of occupational therapy from member organisations. World Federation of Occupational Therapists.

19 The value of exploring the dark side of occupation in pre-registration occupational therapy education, using homelessness as a case study

Miranda Cunningham and Jordan Pace

With acknowledgement to Faith Bowerman (final year student, BSc Hons Occupational Therapy) and Amanda MacArdy (final year student, MSc Pre-Registration Occupational Therapy)

The dark side of occupation in the context of UK curricula

In the United Kingdom, the Royal College of Occupational Therapists (RCOT) (formerly the College of Occupational Therapists (COT)) is the professional body for occupational therapy practitioners. As such, it produces learning and development standards for pre-registration education (RCOT, 2019) which comply with the Minimum Standards for the Education of Occupational Therapists produced by the World Federation of Occupational Therapists (WFOT) (2016). In the minimum standards, WFOT (2016) urges occupational therapists to collaborate with communities who experience social challenges, which might include substance misuse, poverty, or homelessness, to support them to live well. They give a mandate to occupational therapy programmes to focus on building healthy communities through focusing, not only on occupation for health and wellbeing, but also on "occupation as a risk factor for ill health" (WFOT, 2016, p. 14). In the UK, the Royal College of Occupational Therapists Learning and Development Standards do not specify the content of higher education programmes which, arguably, allows for flexibility of provision by institutions (RCOT, 2019). Having said that, RCOT are clear that occupation should be central to the curriculum for pre-registration students (RCOT, 2019). Links are made in the Learning and Development Standards between occupation and health and wellbeing, but there is only a brief mention of engagement in occupations "that are meaningful but harmful" (RCOT, 2019, p. 3). This contrasts with the WFOT standards that suggest a clear link between occupation and ill health (WFOT, 2016). Evidently, there is a need for curricula to include exploration of occupations that link to compromised or ill health, considering this is not explicit in the UK standards. Without this, any exploration of the dark side of occupation is left to the discretion of individual institutions and academic teams.

Why might exploration of the dark side of occupation be important in curricula?

As Twinley (2017) suggests, there are certain occupations that people engage in, which remain unexplored, that challenge the dominant belief that occupations are health-promoting. In complying with standards that assert that occupational therapy's purpose is to transform occupational lives (RCOT, 2019), educators must surely support pre-registration students to understand more fully the nature of human occupation. This means that attention should be paid to human occupation in its diversity, beyond simplistic categories of self-care, productivity, and leisure to include, for example: those that are not health-promoting, occupations to facilitate survival, those that some might consider as antisocial but others find fulfil occupational needs, those that operate as a form of resistance to inequalities, or fulfil purposes other than those currently explored in occupation-based literature.

At the University of Plymouth, both pre-registration BSc and MSc students engage in an occupational studies module that focuses on occupation for promoting the health and wellness of communities. As part of the curriculum students engage in a number of problem-based learning scenarios, one of which is triggered by a photograph of a homeless individual. This thought-provoking photograph is used to stimulate discussion and debate around students' understanding of homelessness, what causes homelessness, and the multiple vulnerabilities that people who experience homelessness are likely to face. Discussion extends to occupational engagement, or the lack thereof, for this population, and exposes students to the variety of occupations that may make up daily life for people who experience homelessness; including many that might fall within the category of the dark side of occupation. In addition, through links with a local homeless residential centre, a number of students are able to gain practice placement experience, actively developing occupational therapy services within the centre itself.

Why is homelessness an appropriate case study for the dark side of occupation?

Homelessness is a complex issue which encompasses multiple challenges; on a daily basis this population may face mental illness, post-traumatic stress, substance misuse, lack of identity and unemployment (Aubry, Klodawsky, & Coulombe, 2011). In 2018, the number of homeless individuals in the UK was around 320,000, a figure that still continues to rise (Shelter, 2018). In London alone, an estimated additional 225,000 "hidden" homeless struggle living in temporary accommodation (Fransham & Dorling, 2018). Following the Coronavirus pandemic that started in 2019, homelessness – as a global issue – will change. However, regardless of the time and context, the daily struggles that people who experience homelessness face are not limited to a lack of permanent residence. The Homeless Reduction Act (2017) highlights the importance of current and integrative legislation to prevent and alleviate the challenges of homelessness. Third-sector organisations strive to provide for the needs of the people who experience homelessness, providing housing, skills, education, food, drug, and health services (Buckingham, 2012).

Erikson (1959) wrote about the importance of forming an identity to consolidate role, goals, and values to develop an intrinsic sense of self. For many people, positive identity formation can be developed through engagement in meaningful occupations (Cunningham, 2016). For people who experience homelessness, deprivation of occupational opportunities can lead to social exclusion and an inability to partake in economic, cultural, and social aspects of wider society; this contributes to high-risk behaviours and impaired psychological and physical health (Watson, Crawley, & Kane, 2016). Those experiencing mental illness, in particular, experience a lack of meaningful connection and belonging due to discrimination and stigma (Le Boutillier & Croucher, 2010). The homeless population is frequently forced to engage in survival occupations such as finding shelter, theft, prostitution, or substance abuse (Illman, Spence, O'Campo, & Kirsh, 2013). While such occupations can still carry meaning, most are adopted simply to preserve life, with the experience of homelessness placing considerable physical and psychological demands on people (Cunningham & Slade, 2017).

It is crucial, however, not to overlook the significance of occupations which oppose preconceptions of a "healthy" lifestyle. If occupation is to be understood as central to developing personal identity, abstinence from occupations that might be considered on the dark side, as they are unexplored, may result in occupational deficit for homeless individuals (Wasmuth, Crabtree, & Scott, 2014). For example, evidence shows that while drug use can be detrimental to overall health and wellbeing, it can still hold value and meaning to an individual. As a co-occupation it can foster opportunities to connect with other users; this can lead to formation of identity, values and personal role within a group (Wasmuth, Crabtree, & Scott, 2014). It can be argued that social connectedness is critical to a sense of belonging, purpose, and meaning (Cruwys, Haslam, Dingle, Haslam, & Jetten, 2014). While some find identity gained through engaging in occupations that might be considered on the dark side, others may experience identity loss. Assigned terms such as "junkie" or "alcoholic" can devalue or "spoil" an established sense of identity (Dingle, Cruwys, & Frings, 2015). While it can be easy to dismiss occupations that may not align with broader society's values, such a mono-polistic approach would arguably be contrary to the holistic nature of our discipline and should be avoided.

Reflections on students' experiences of exposure to the dark side of occupation during placement

For people who experience homelessness, engagement in occupation is a complex phenomenon, situated in their own particular cultural, political, and economic context. When students engage in practice placement experiences in the homeless shelter an initial period of adjustment occurs, which is typical of many placement settings. However, in addition, there is considerable and continued exposure to the dark side of occupation. This placement experience allows students to realise the complexity of occupation, perhaps more so than in other, more traditional settings. Students list the occupations that they are aware are occurring which fall outside typical ideas of health-giving occupation, which include: misuse of prescription medication, use of "hard" and "soft" street drugs, dealing drugs, running drugs, misuse of alcohol, high levels of gaming including video gaming, sexual favours, begging, and violent behaviour.

Prior to placement, students might describe their understanding of the dark side of occupation from an academic viewpoint only; some admit to having a fairly sheltered upbringing where prior contact with the dark side of occupation may have been limited, which may reflect a lack of diversity in the cohort. Understanding of the concept can also be limited to perceiving these occupations as non-health-promoting. However, placement experience has helped students to view occupations in context and to appreciate the potential for positive impact; for example, students observed residents engaging in gaming as a leisure occupation – facilitating social connections – and as a means of restoration, in an otherwise occupationally deprived environment. In contrast, students also witnessed first-hand the negative impact of gaming, when it became addictive, impacting on routines, with residents staying up all night to engage in online competitions, missing meals, and going into debt to buy in-game purchases.

Students are aware that many residents use substances as a coping mechanism for anxiety and depression. Whilst alcohol consumption is legal in the UK, possession and use of marijuana is illegal, although police forces sometimes take a more lenient view of marijuana possession for personal use. Students have expressed that service users confide in them about their substance use because they are viewed as likely to be less punitive than hostel staff. It is not unusual for students to be viewed differently by people who use services; however, this situation puts students in an uncomfortable position, as a bridge between residents and staff.

In this setting, students experience a very different daily life to the one that they may be used to. Students are witness to occupational injustices, including residents' experiences of occupational deprivation and alienation. There is a perception of a lack of balance in meaningful occupation amongst the residents that is on a scale that students are not usually exposed to. Boredom is significant, which has manifested in either very long occupational "drop in" sessions run by students, or impulsive behaviour where residents very much live in the moment. Students observe how certain occupations take precedence over all others, including attending the job centre, getting money, and collecting prescriptions. This supports students' understanding of occupational priorities for people and how these may differ from staff or hostel expectations.

Perhaps the greatest dilemma cited by students, in respect of the placement, relates to their position as healthcare professionals in training. They are acutely aware of their code of ethics and responsibilities in relation to their professional conduct. This can present barriers in relation to discussions of everyday occupations with residents, which often include substance use; impacting on their ability to build rapport, trust, and understanding as genuinely empathetic and interested human beings. Some personally significant occupations that residents engage in are not only detrimental to health; in the case of many substances, their use is illegal. Whilst students articulate their ability to consider substance use as an occupation from an occupational science perspective, they are unsure of how to deal with disclosures of substance use in practice. Students acknowledge and value support given in supervision and recognise their professional duties outlined in codes of ethics (i.e. Health and Care Professions Council (HCPC), 2016). However, this picture is complex because students perceive hostel staff members to be conflicted about the residents' use of substances. It is common, as part of the support provided by professional drug services and residential service staff, for users to be supplied with sharps bins as a contribution to safe use of drugs. Attitudes to this may also be affected by the fact that some staff in services may be in recovery themselves and, therefore, aware of the value of safe use as a part of the recovery journey. This mix of perspectives is a novel experience for students who struggle to deal with their own opposing rationales when confronted by residents who openly disclose substance misuse. Students do not wish to advocate for non-health-promoting behaviours (and contravene professional codes of ethics) whilst attempting to build rapport with fellow occupational beings, recognising the value of substance misuse – in the short term at least – as a coping mechanism, or as an occupation that provides connection and routine.

These blurred boundaries can lead to fear on all sides. Students express fear in relation to discussing these occupations in case they might be "struck off" their professional register. Students also observe how some residents disengage from interventions led by staff because they do not want to be open about their occupations, fuelled by stigma and a desire to continue engaging with substances. Students also feel that residents avoid visiting the doctor for fear of being found out as actively using.

The HCPC regulates a number of healthcare professions in the UK, including occupational therapists. They publish standards for registrants and also guidance on conduct and ethics for students (HCPC, 2016). Whilst the guidance "does not provide answers to every situation you may face" (HCPC, 2016, p. 7), it is clear that if any confidential information arises that might impact the wellbeing of someone, this should be discussed. In addition, appropriate local and educational policies should be followed (HCPC, 2016). The placement setting has a policy of "harm reduction" in relation to licit or illicit substance use where a number of strategies are employed, including safer use, managed use, and abstinence. Openness and sharing of information is encouraged in the setting, which adopts comparable rules in relation to confidentiality.

The harm reduction philosophy follows a number of principles that should allow students some flexibility in relation to working with residents who use substances. For example, harm reduction acknowledges that substance use is a part of life, and rather than ignoring it, or condemning users, healthcare professionals should work to minimise harmful effects (Harm Reduction Coalition, n.d.). Unfortunately, there is evidence amongst health professionals that not all attitudes are this progressive (Biley, 2006). It would be naive to suspect that only those graduates who obtain jobs in certain settings, for example substance misuse teams or mental health, are likely to encounter substance misuse, or other occupations that might be described as on the dark side. A study by Kelleher (2007) found that as many as 28% of people attending hospital emergency departments in Ireland had a substance misuse-related illness or injury. Additionally, there is a risk that healthcare professionals themselves develop substance misuse disorders (Sørensen, 2019). Negative attitudes to substance users can adversely impact on care to the extent that Kelleher (2007) is recommending better preparation of undergraduate healthcare professionals. This study was further supported by a later systematic review (van Boekel, Brouwers, van Weeghel, & Garretsen, 2013) which concluded that negative attitudes are common amongst healthcare professionals and can reduce patients' feelings of empowerment and subsequent health outcomes.

Conclusion

There is a clear need for an overt tackling of issues in relation to the dark side of occupation, in the curriculum, beyond theorising and into practice. We express this need because, in our experience, pre-registration students must be equipped with the skills to manage the situations described in an open, non-judgemental way, and without breaching standards, whilst respecting confidentiality, as far as is possible within their remit. Using real-life case studies and varied placement settings allows students opportunities to confront and work through important issues, particularly in relation to disclosure of information from clients and appropriate actions in relation to codes of ethics. Having an opportunity to explore substance use as an occupation should support students to develop a more nuanced understanding of human occupation and contextual factors that influence it. This is particularly powerful when supporting students to develop a critical perspective on the nature of substance use beyond individual motivations to some of the wider socio-economic factors that influence it. Harm reduction as a philosophy is consistent with an occupational perspective on substance use; increasing knowledge of these strategies amongst pre-registration occupational therapy students will support a more integrated and compassionate approach to developing knowledge and practice in relation to the dark side of occupation.

References

Aubry, T., Klodawsky, F., & Coulombe, D. (2011). Comparing the housing trajectories of different classes within a diverse homeless population. *American Journal of Community Psychology, 49*(1–2), pp. 142–155. doi:10.1007/s10464-011-9444-z.

Biley, F.C. (2006). The arts, literature and the attraction paradigm: Changing attitudes towards substance misuse service users. *Journal of Substance Use, 11*(1), pp. 11–21. https://doi.org/10.1080/14659890412331334400.

Buckingham, H. (2012). Capturing diversity: A typology of third sector organisations' responses to contracting based on empirical evidence from homelessness services. *Journal of Social Policy, 41*(3), pp. 569–689. https://doi.org/10.1017/S0047279412000086.

Cruwys, T., Haslam, S.A., Dingle, G.A., Haslam, C., & Jetten, J. (2014). Depression and social identity: An integrative review. *Personality and Social Psychology Review, 18*(3), pp. 215–238. doi:10.1177/1088868314523839.

Cunningham, M.J. (2016). Broadening understandings of occupational identity: Illustrations from a research study of homeless adults. In D. Sakellariou & N. Pollard (Eds.), *Occupational therapies without borders: Integrating justice with practice* (pp. 118–130). Edinburgh: Elsevier.

Cunningham, M., & Slade, A. (2017). Exploring the lived experience of homelessness from an occupational perspective. *Scandinavian Journal of Occupational Therapy, 26*(1), pp. 19–32. www.tandfonline.com/doi/abs/10.1080/11038128.2017.1304572.

Dingle, G., Cruwys, T., & Frings, D. (2015). Social identities as pathways into and out of addiction. *Frontiers in Psychology, 6*, 1795. https://doi.org/10.3389/fpsyg.2015.01795.

Erikson, E.H. (1959). *Identity and the life cycle: Selected papers.* Oxford: International Universities Press.

Fransham, M., & Dorling, D. (2018). Homelessness and public health. *British Medical Journal, 360*: k214. https://doi.org/10.1136/bmj.k214.

Harm Reduction Coalition (n.d.). Principles of harm reduction. Retrieved from https://harmreduction.org/about-us/principles-of-harm-reduction/.

Health and Care Professions Council (2016). Guidance on conduct and ethics for students. Retrieved from www.hcpc-uk.org/globalassets/resources/guidance/guidance-on-conduct-and-ethics-for-students.pdf.

Homeless Reduction Act (2017). London: The Stationary Office.

Illman, S.C., Spence, S., O'Campo, P.J., & Kirsh, B.H. (2013). Exploring the occupations of homeless adults living with mental illnesses in Toronto. *Canadian Journal of Occupational Therapy*, *80*(4), pp. 215–223. doi:10.1177/0008417413 506555.

Kelleher, S. (2007). Health care professionals' knowledge and attitudes regarding substance use and substance users. *Accident and Emergency Nursing*, *15*(3), pp. 161–165. https://doi.org/10.1016/j.aaen.2007.05.005.

Le Boutillier, C., & Croucher, A. (2010). Social inclusion and mental health. *British Journal of Occupational Therapy*, *73*(3), pp. 136–139. https://doi.org/10.4276/03080 2210X12682330090578.

Royal College of Occupational Therapists (2019). *Learning and development standards for pre-registration education*. London: Royal College of Occupational Therapists. Retrieved from www.rcot.co.uk/practice-resources/rcot-publications/learning-and-development-standards-pre-registration-education.

Shelter (2018, 22 November). 320,000 people in Britain are now homeless, as numbers keep rising. Retrieved from https://england.shelter.org.uk/media/press_releases/articles/320,000_people_in_britain_are_now_homeless,_as_numbers_keep_rising.

Sørensen, J.K. (2019). How physicians' professional socialisation and social technologies may affect colleagues in substance use disorders. *Addiction Research & Theory*, *27*(2), pp. 104–113, doi:10.1080/16066359.2018.1457654.

Twinley, R. (2017). The dark side of occupation. In K. Jacobs & N. MacRae (Eds.), *Occupational therapy essentials for clinical competence* (3rd ed., pp. 29–36). Thorofare, NJ: Slack.

van Boekel, L., Brouwers, E.P.M., van Weeghel, J., & Garretsen, H.F.L. (2013). Stigma among health professionals towards patients with substance use disorders and its consequences for healthcare delivery: Systematic review. *Drug and Alcohol Dependence*, *31*(1–2), pp. 23–35. doi:10.1016/j.drugalcdep.2013.02.018.

Wasmuth, S., Crabtree, J.L., & Scott, P.J. (2014). Exploring addiction-as-occupation. *British Journal of Occupational Therapy*, *77*(12), pp. 605–613. https://doi.org/10.4276/030802214X14176260335264.

Watson, J., Crawley, J., & Kane, D. (2016). Social exclusion, health and hidden homelessness. *Public Health*, *139*, pp. 96–102. doi:10.1016/j.puhe.2016.05.017.

World Federation of Occupational Therapists (2016). Minimum standards for the education of occupational therapists. Retrieved from www.wfot.org/resources/new-minimum-standards-for-the-education-of-occupational-therapists-2016-e-copy.

20 The dark side of occupation

A conversation of our evolution and our future

Rebecca Twinley, Karen Jacobs, and Channine Clarke

Initial remarks from Rebecca

Very practically, when a profession like occupational therapy declares it "takes a 'whole-person approach' to both mental and physical health and wellbeing and enables individuals to achieve their full potential" (Royal College of Occupational Therapists, 2019), there needs to be genuine consideration of the whole person. That is, I (Bex) stand by my assertion that:

> In an attempt to truly become more holistic practitioners, theorists, researchers and educators we need to not just be aware of, but also strive to understand, the dark side of occupation. We must continue to consider the subjectivity of human occupation and an individual's unique lived experience ... It is crucial our analysis, construction, comprehension and critique of occupation continue to develop and evolve.
>
> (Twinley, 2013, p. 303)

To do so, there is a critical need to address our position in terms of being a globally relevant and inclusive profession, as Whalley Hammell stressed:

> Surely, the occupational therapy profession can be positioned to have a relevant and significant global impact if we build from the strength of our diversity, and work together towards ensuring that all people, regardless of difference, have the capabilities (i.e. both the abilities and the opportunities) to engage in occupations that contribute to their own well-being and the well-being of their communities, as is their right.
>
> (2019, p. 13)

As creator of the theoretical concept of the dark side of occupation, I am very aware that I formulated this in my specific contexts (i.e. geographical, cultural, sociopolitical, economic). As editor of this text, I really wanted to include and present diverse, cross-cultural perspectives, especially because the whole intent of my concept was to prompt people to consider and explore the "gaps in existing knowledge and identify what has been overlooked, obscured, omitted and assumed" (Whalley Hammell, 2019, p. 13). Like much occupational science scholarship, the dark side of occupation emerged – as a concept – in the UK. It is, therefore, very likely that any emergence of contributions from non-English-speaking countries could be "frequently hampered by diverse barriers to global collaboration, knowledge dissemination, and inclusion in international dialogue" (Magalhães et al., 2019). When inviting contributors, I largely had to rely upon my professional network and colleagues. I also needed to invite people who either had awareness of, had cited, or whose work was akin to, the dark side of occupation. I sought a range of contributors who could write a chapter for inclusion in one of the four sections. Moreover, of course, as an endeavour contracted by a UK-based branch of a global publisher, contributors who can write in English were sought. All of this places constraints on the text, especially in terms of presenting wider international and diverse perspectives. I am deeply grateful to those contributors to this text and we have, together, presented some ground-breaking, practice-changing international perspectives. I would wish for future endeavours to embrace more globally diverse perspectives. Our world is rich with diversity and we should be learning more about our global colleagues and their work. I believe I would speak for us all in saying that what we hope this text has achieved is to prompt you to think about occupations as they relate to you, and how they may relate to the rest of the world.

Initial remarks from Karen

I first met Bex when the OT4OT team was scheduling speakers for OT24Vx2014: A World of Health and Well Being held 3–4 November 2014. Bex was invited to provide a virtual presentation entitled, " 'Everyone is a moon': The dark side of occupation". This was my first time learning about the construct of "the dark side of occupation" which Bex coined. In 2015, I recall inviting Bex to write a chapter on the dark side of occupation. She was happy to accept this invitation and "The Dark Side of Occupation" became Chapter 3 in the 3rd edition of *Occupational Therapy Essentials for Clinical Competency* (Jacobs & MacRae, 2017). "The Dark Side of Occupation" continues to be a well-read and thought-provoking chapter, but it needed a larger avenue for discussion of this important topic. Bex and I discussed this in a podcast (see https://podcasts.apple.com/us/podcast/lifestyle-by-design-helping-you-solve-everyday-challenges/id1360274216), and this has occurred within the pages of this text.

The contribution of the dark side of occupation for theory

The chapters in this section responded to the challenge of critically considering the dark side of occupation as a theoretical concept and from a theoretical stance; they have therefore grappled with issues such as the terminological debate that has ensued, and they provide some powerful and necessary context to the intent and subject matter of this text in its entirety.

Hocking (Chapter 2) offered a tangible overview of the limited occupational science literature which has provided in-depth insights into some of the occupations which have, otherwise, remained largely unexplored. The labelling of other people's occupations, and the predominant Western worldview regarding use of terms, is borne out in her discussion of the five identified common features from the literature that explores occupations characterised as unhealthy, damaging, deviant, or disrupted.

Reflecting historically, as McKay (Chapter 3) has done, in terms of the position of the occupational therapy profession, it is useful to be mindful of factors that have created and contributed to the lack of address of occupations that are not meaningful or healthful. This is part of the profession's history and, therefore, represents the underlying theoretical assumptions that were made as occupational therapy emerged and developed. By considering the dark side of occupation, it is these assumptions that are challenged (and some that need dispelling) so that our theoretical underpinnings evolve to truly reflect contemporary practice issues, which concedes the need to appreciate the absolute range and diversity of occupations. Considering this potential, Hart (Chapter 4) examined the capacity of our existing "occupational lens" when we are, increasingly, working with people with diverse occupational lives. It is asserted that there is a need to attend to our professional positionality, and to be critical in order to fully "see" occupation. Hart's discussion notes the domination of key theoretical models of occupational therapy practice, posing the critique that perhaps these Western-derived models are too simple, or too prescriptive, to apply to phenomena that are complex, uncomfortable, and unknown.

The consensus is such that theory regarding the dark side of occupation is emerging and evolving. One lesser realised phenomenon of contributing to this development and evolution is evident from Whiteford and Haddad's chapter (Chapter 5) – that of the need for Haddad's identity to remain anonymous due to the political climate and tensions. In striving to explore the hidden, the silenced, the invisible, their contribution is evidence in and of itself of the need for invisibility experienced by some colleagues and commentators; people whose work develops and contributes to gaining a more informed and diversely rich occupational perspective, but who are personally and professionally at risk from doing so. Additionally, their chapter is a constructive example of how politics influences theory, highlighting the need for theory to develop as political forces and tensions

184 Rebecca Twinley et al.

change; for we cannot remove ourselves as occupational beings from the political context within which we live.

Reflective questions

- What occupations do you regularly confront that have known health risks but have not been apparent in discourse or theory regarding occupation?
- What occupations do you pursue that you hide (perhaps to varying degrees, depending on your social group and environment) to avoid judgement by others?
- Which theoretical perspectives have influenced you and your thinking? Have they prompted you to consider occupations that may not necessarily link to health or wellbeing?
- As a theoretical concept, the dark side of occupation has very practical implications for those studying or practising in the profession of occupational therapy and the discipline of occupational science. Can you think about what some of these implications are for you?

The contribution of the dark side of occupation for research

The research section of this collection includes examples from studies conducted that present aspects of the subjective experience of occupations which needed uncovering and which have, subsequently, been explored from an occupational perspective. These contributions are representative of bold and brave research endeavours by people who have, for instance, faced challenges, overcome barriers, and dealt with traumatic content in order to address some of the gaps in evidence regarding the dark side of occupation. Issues such as homelessness have, thankfully, generated increasing attention, as evident by the very fact that Boland, Marshall, and Westover's chapter (Chapter 6) is the result of their collaboration. From what is acknowledged to be a Western perspective, they have successfully proposed how the value of an occupational perspective of the occupational lives of homeless persons needs to be recognised at a policy and organisational level; to do so, they assert the dark side – that is, the unacknowledged aspects of their occupational experiences – must be uncovered and more fully understood.

Findings from research can have significance for practice; Luck's (Chapter 7) exploration of smoking highlights how feelings of shame and guilt might impede the therapeutic relationship, in terms of "admitting" to doing things viewed – largely – as unhealthy or undesirable. This is suggestive of issues faced in addressing the dark side of occupation, especially considering tobacco smoking – which is understood to be regarded by many non-smokers as unpleasant – is not necessarily a sensitive or uncomfortable topic; certainly not in comparison to the subject matter of Mercer's chapter (Chapter 8), in which she presents a single case study to highlight the complex reasons, meanings, and experience of self-defeating occupations. This work is a window into how a person subjectively experiences something extremely private that is, ordinarily, hidden. Research that seeks to reveal aspects of hidden or invisible experience is paramount to enhancing our understanding of the dark side of occupation and will have both benefits and implications for practice.

An issue close to Rebecca's heart and very being is the public health problem of rape and sexual assault. At the time of conducting her PhD on the topic of woman-to-woman rape, Rebecca found just one author (Froehlich, 1992) who had explored adult sexual victimisation from an occupational perspective in order to outline the role occupational therapists could have. As an outcome of previous collaborative work, Rebecca was keen to include a contribution from Taylor (Chapter 9), who is a recognised expert in the field of child and adult sexual victimisation. Hence, Taylor's chapter incorporates her knowledge and experience in criminology and forensic science to discuss an under-explored issue. This chapter is evidence of the contribution to our occupational perspective that non-occupational therapist occupational scientists can provide, as it highlights the work-related disadvantages created as a consequence of childhood sexual abuse. As such, this is an exemplary piece of research that has pushed boundaries in order to illuminate some of the impacts of sexual trauma on people's occupations.

Reflective questions

- How can researchers contribute to decolonising methodologies and thus to ensuring the dominant trends no longer hinder our understanding of the complexity and array of occupations?
- Do current ethical considerations for research in occupational therapy and occupational science need to encompass the possibility, likelihood even, of research that will propose to explore professionally challenging, risky, illegal, or highly traumatic issues and occupations?
- Will occupational therapy and occupational science professionals have the courage and obtain the support needed to investigate challenging, risky, illegal, or highly traumatic issues and occupations?

The contribution of the dark side of occupation for practice

We suggest it is paramount to ask the people you work with and for, what it is they want, need, hope for in terms of talking about the dark side of occupation. An essential question to pose is: How can we talk about the dark side of occupation in practice? The truth is, there is no clear-cut answer. In his chapter, Greber (Chapter 10) tackles the very practical (or bottom line) issue that occupational therapists and, indeed, all health and care professionals will face when working with people who choose to engage in illicit, immoral, and health-compromising occupations; the reasoning skills necessary to do so are discussed. A constructive example of work in which ethical dilemmas are faced is found in Nhunzvi and Galvaan's chapter (Chapter 11), in which they present findings from a narrative inquiry into the journey of recovery from substance abuse among young adult Zimbabwean men. Substance use and abuse is explored and understood as an occupation – one which can change over time, alongside other occupations that can facilitate or inhibit recovery.

Further, as an insight into what has been done and worked well in practice, Cowan and Sørlie (Chapter 12) shared their experiences of introducing the dark side of occupation into a weekly occupation-focused group with service users in an occupational therapy-led intensive day service for people with longstanding eating disorders. We learn about the way the concept was utilised to change and improve upon practice, as they also give an instructive example of occupation-focused practice in an acute setting.

Realistically, we know there are so many constraints on practice (and we mean before the Coronavirus pandemic impacted upon us as it has) and it is the responsibility of all of us to determine practical and possible ways in which the dark side of occupation can enter into discussions. We need to consider the environments we work in and the extent to which they are conducive to having these (potentially) less comfortable or, even, more open discussions. Morris' and Tyminski's chapters (Chapter 13 and 14) are examples of efforts to change practice. Morris explicitly shows how her framework to position occupational engagement – developed through her doctoral research with men living in a secure forensic unit – could be used to illuminate the dark side of occupation in people's lives. In terms of assessment tools, Tyminski presents a newly developed version of the Activity Card Sort (Baum & Edwards, 2008) that could be used with homeless people. This achievement marks the beginning of developments that will see our occupational lens shift to seeing, as Hart discussed, occupation more in its totality. We note these examples are based largely on a "working age" adult population and should not detract from the need to attend to the dark side of occupation in childhood and adolescence (including, for instance, practice with children experiencing obesity) and in older adulthood (such as risk-taking).

Reflective questions

- Is there a need to include the dark side of occupation in ethical codes of conduct and practice?
- What do you consider to be the taken for granted views about the "unhealthy" occupation of substance use?

- For those of you reading this from a Western perspective and position, what have you learned from insight into the experiential occupational nature of substance use in an African context?
- Can you discuss linkages between understanding the dark side of occupation and promoting recovery from substance use disorders?
- To what extent do you think occupations perceived or judged by many to be "risky" can be survival and social inclusion pillars?
- What are the ethical dilemmas involved in practice that is informed by knowledge of the dark side of occupation?
- In what ways can we take a trauma-informed approach to our work?
- How can we develop our interviewing skills, models, assessment, and evaluation tools?

The contribution of the dark side of occupation for education

Collectively, the inclusion of newly qualified (Agyemang and Pace) and educator (Ennals, Nastasi, Di Tommaso, and Cunningham) voices has really evaluated the necessity to understand the meaning offered by health-compromising occupations. Agyemang's (Chapter 15) assertion that it is necessary for students to test the robustness of the founding notions of the occupational therapy profession, and to look at the complex consideration of the relationship between occupation and health, must be noted by educators – especially those involved in curriculum design and development; the chapters by Nastasi, Di Tommaso, and Cunningham and Pace are a suggested starting place if this is something you seek to achieve.

Nastasi's (Chapter 17) proposal of the way in which students can be facilitated to learn about the dark side of occupation, by exploring the interaction between a person, their occupations, and the environment, shows how small but necessary changes can bring about a more holistic teaching and learning experience. Likewise, Cunningham and Pace's (Chapter 19) reflections on teaching and learning about an aspect of the dark side of occupation through a case study are a helpful way to see how students can test ideas in the classroom or in supervision, whilst tackling difficult issues in practice, such as substance use. Di Tommaso's contribution (Chapter 18) provides further evidence for integrating the dark side of occupation into curricula, as she found two cohorts of final year students gained a deeper understanding of theoretical knowledge. The fact her students felt more prepared for future practice indicates a need to develop work in this area.

Bringing us back to the dark side of occupation as something which we have all experienced, or very likely do experience, Ennals' chapter (Chapter 16) highlights considerations for educators and students alike and should make us all mindful of the effect that perceived stress can have upon our subjective experience of occupations.

Reflective questions

- How can your teaching activities be relevant to the problems of people with whom your students will work?
- What is your level of preparedness to discuss the dark side of occupation? Do you, or can you, open up conversation about lesser discussed occupations that could be important, valued, meaningful, or necessary in people's lives?
- Where do you stand ethically and morally if people need to talk about or want to engage in occupations that are, socially, viewed to push against the acceptable norms, or that violate laws?
- If you agree there is a need to examine, understand, and teach about the overlooked dark side of occupation, how might you achieve this?
- Is there a need to include the dark side of occupation in pre-registration (educational programme) curriculum standards for occupational therapy?

Rebecca's concluding thoughts: it's "part of our evolution"

I have Bonnie Kennedy to thank for making the comment "Perhaps you should view this as part of our evolution" to someone at a conference who was at odds with the inclusion of the word "dark" in my concept's name. I guess it had not fully occurred to me that, just as I read and learn from the legacy of scholarly works, the discussions that have started to take place are already shaping and redefining our understanding of occupation. Therefore, regardless of personally-held beliefs or assumptions about the name "the dark side of occupation", the concept itself has already contributed toward the inevitable and much needed evolution of the theoretical underpinnings of professions and disciplines that study human occupation. Having collaborated and enjoyed engaging with people from disciplines such as criminology, psychology, sociology, and disability studies, I very much believe an occupational perspective has much to offer those other professions and disciplines which seek to understand people and their occupations. Additionally, I concur with Hammell and Iwama's (2012) call for theorists to "commit to rigorous efforts to seek out diverse global perspectives – that have tended to be overlooked, unacknowledged, or discounted – both to achieve inclusivity and relevance and to counter theoretical tendencies to colonialism and imperialism" (Hammell, 2017, p. 52).

The most appropriate place to implement changes to thinking, which translates then into theory, practice, and research, is with those people who are new to learning about occupation: students, and not just occupational therapy or science students. As discussed earlier, I feel strongly that an occupational perspective can contribute to those other professions and disciplines that aim to understand people in terms of occupation, nature, behaviour, motivation, achievement, culture, and lived experience. This also demands that academics/teachers/educators need to contest awkward assumptions that are present as a result of the historical background of occupational therapy. There is, therefore, the potential to face difficult situations, especially with peers and colleagues who are less inclined or motivated to evolve with the times; specifically, this means challenging the dominant intellectual orientation that informed the development of the profession and subsequent training. Globally, occupational therapy training and education has, to varying extents, been standardised; the very nature of standardisation (achieved mostly through Minimum Curriculum Standards) demands conformity and has produced academic colonialism. This means those involved in occupational therapy education taking place in the dominant (Western) centre of knowledge-production (such as the UK, USA, and Canada) are at an advantage compared to their peers working in knowledge-dependent states (Shih, 2009). This privilege is evident in research endeavours whereby anything not regarded as from dominant knowledge-producing efforts is othered, as Biermann highlights from work that has: "encouraged Indigenous intellectuals to continue resisting dominant approaches to academic knowledge production and to develop their own methodologies based on anti-colonial paradigms" (2001, p. 386).

All of this, this need to evolve, is because of the people we work with and for. When it comes to occupational therapy practice, we need to always be thinking of ways to survive as well as flourish. As experts in occupation, I cannot see how we will achieve this if we do not pay (more) attention to addressing occupations in people's lives that shape who they are, what they do, who they do it with, how they are perceived, why they are doing it, where, for how long, what it meant, and how it felt – those beyond the safe and comfortable occupations that persist to be categorised into the three domains of self-care, productivity, and leisure.

Thinking about now and the future: it's beyond our imagination

We do not yet know what we do not yet know. Obvious. Nevertheless, this obviousness is verification for the necessity for our understanding of occupations and of people, groups, communities, populations, and societies to evolve with the passing of time and the changes it will bring. For many of us, within the space of one week, our worlds changed as the Coronavirus (Covid-19) pandemic spread and led to changes in the way we worked, practised, connected, communicated, and lived; this was unexpected and demanded a great amount of adaptation, resilience, respect, trust, effort, and humour, even. We must be diligent in addressing the dark side of occupation in a timely manner. With this, we need people who will lead on challenging assumptions, ideas, and theories so that the understanding and use of occupation is always deemed and perceived to be contemporary: appropriate and responsive to people's wants and needs at the time, and in the place, these are experienced. We need agents of change who are committed long term to exploring the dark side of occupation. There are so many challenges and circumstances that can lead to the dark side of occupation occurring that we need to more wholly address. To elucidate, we use five tables (20.1–20.5) to present examples of where efforts could be focused, as outlined here:

- In terms of challenging assumptions, Table 20.1 shows some concepts we feel need more consideration and scrutiny.
- Table 20.2 gives some examples of daily occupations that remain under-addressed. Many of these were gathered via a real-time voting tool used during an event Rebecca hosted in February 2020 with an occupational therapy audience.
- Then, there are contemporary concerns affecting many people, groups, communities, populations, and societies (Table 20.3). One current concern as we write this chapter is the Coronavirus pandemic. The impact this global crisis will have had on people's subjective experiences of occupations can only be speculated on at this time. In what ways might we need to learn to adapt our occupations and our work in preparation for any such future epidemics or pandemics?
- There are many significant biographical disruptions (Bury, 1982) where we need to far better focus our efforts. This warrants acknowledgement that "a biographical disruption can be a disruptive but potentially important experience; one which might instigate a person's reassessment of their norms, values, priorities, identity, and choices in relation to their occupations" (Twinley, 2016, p. 83). As Table 20.4 portrays, disruptions can lead people to experience varying "states" of being and wellbeing; we need to better understand these, such as trauma and boredom.
- With the expansion of occupational therapy into new, diverse, and emerging roles, therapists are ideally placed to start open and honest discussions with the wider population about occupations that may be considered meaningful to them but unhealthy, harmful, or unnecessary by others. Table 20.5 provides some examples of the types of diverse settings occupational therapists are increasingly working in and the dark side of occupation that they will need to discuss with their clients, colleagues, and commissioners. In doing so, they will be able to highlight the valuable contribution they and occupational therapy can make outside of traditional health and social care services. The example of gender identity services illustrates how the dark side of occupation is not just about the detrimental or harmful occupations people perform; it is also about exploring or seeking to understand people's engagement in occupations that they feel must be performed in secret, or the experience of finding new occupations during, for instance, the process of transitioning.

Table 20.1 A table to show the challenges to existing concepts and assumptions

Co-occupation	Occupational justice	Occupational balance	General assumptions that occupations are:
Can this lead to frustration (i.e. when it occurs between people and their carer or a support worker)? Can it be overwhelming? What about when it is enforced?	What does this "look like" during a global pandemic like Coronavirus (Covid-19)? Can we talk about this, let alone strive for this, for a global majority when people experience infringements or complete violations of their human rights?	Does the global political and socioeconomic climate prevent the very possibility of achieving some sense of this?	• Meaningful • Purposeful • Empowering • Have a positive contribution to health and wellbeing • Safe • Healthful • Enjoyable • Restorative • Therapeutic

Table 20.2 A table to show the daily or regularly-experienced occupations that remain under-addressed

Sex, dating, and intimacy	Religious or spiritual practice or "doing"	Survival occupations	Addiction
• Being, doing, and becoming "sexually attractive" • Sexual desires • Sexual avoidance • Sexual "perversions" • Masturbation • Dogging • Swinging • Polyamory • Sex and disability • Sex as work • Impact of acute or chronic health problems	• Diverse experiences of religious doing • Spirituality as a key component in some people's lives • Changes to practices as a result of, for instance, enforced isolation during a global pandemic • Lack of associated multi-faith research (see Eyres, Bannigan, & Letherby, 2019)	The shame, secrecy, stigma, guilt, or embarrassment people report to feel when they were engaging in occupations more privately, secretively, as a way to cope or to manage	• Mobile/smart phones • Gaming • Caffeine • Gambling • Sex • Substances • Pornography • Shopping • Exercise • Food (obesity, eating disorders, being a "feeder") • Self-improvement or enhancement treatments and surgeries (i.e. plastic surgery, Botox, tanning)

Table 20.3 A table to show contemporary concerns for occupational therapists and occupational scientists

Social media	Crime and criminality	Prejudice, discrimination, oppression, and exclusion	Health epidemics or pandemics
• Effects on relationships (i.e. between parents and children) • Bullying • Harassment • Stalking • Sexual perpetration • Social withdrawal • Contribution to feelings of (low) self-esteem • Provoking anxiety and/or depression • Impact on sleep	• Its role in giving meaning, status, power • Contribution to formation and enactment of roles and identity	• Ableism • Ageism • Anti-Semitism • Cissexism • Classism • Colonialism • Colourism • Ethnocentrism • Healthism • Heterosexism • Homophobia • Imperialism • Islamophobia • Racism • Sexism • Sizeism • Transphobia • Weightism • Xenophobia	• Such as coronavirus (Covid-19) (2019) • Looting • Stockpiling • Effects of distancing and/or isolation, including on occupations and on experiences such as no escape from ongoing interpersonal violence and abuse • Protests • Rise in racism, criminal, and malicious acts • Impact of restricted finances, religious practices, educational and vocational pursuits, leisure, travel, entertainment, sports and exercise, intimate and other relations and relationships

Table 20.4 A table to show biographical disruptions people experience

Things people do when in different "states"	Changes to health status	People affected by collective trauma following (for instance)	Rape, sexual assault, and abuse
• Anger • Boredom • Elation • Flow • Frustration • Bereaved • Amusement • Contentment • Excitement • Contempt • Embarrassment • Relief • Pride • Guilt • Traumatised and post-traumatised	• Diagnosis of acute or chronic condition • Late diagnosis of something such as autism, as Rebecca experienced in 2019 • Prognosis • Improved health • Dramatic self-change	• Terrorist attacks • Environmental disasters, including bush fires, flooding, and earthquakes • Living under political repressions, such as the Apartheid regime • Living in war zones • Genocide (including survivors of the Holocaust) • Global pandemics	• One-time event • Repeated occurrence • Across the lifespan

Table 20.5 A table to show the dark side of occupation in diverse settings

Prisons	Areas of conflict/ combat/disaster/ pandemics	State-funded schools	Gender identity development services (clinics)
• Drug dealing • Violent acts • Abuses of power • Sexual abuse • Exploitation • Deprivation/ solitary confinement • Suicide • Reoffending/ learning new crimes • Manipulation • Escape attempts • Development of new skills and interests	• Looting after natural disasters • Stockpiling • Fraudulent compensation claims • Terrorist activity • Gang activity • Illegal protests/ demonstrations	• Bullying • Non-attendance • Drug dealing • Abuse • Eating and staying healthy • Impact of problems in home environment, or turbulent relationships with peers	• Avoidance of occupations (due to fear of other people's reactions) • Substance abuse • Sex work • Effects of stigma and discrimination • Coming out as transgender • Transitioning • Learning new occupations • Secret occupations (e.g. cross-dressing)

Issues to consider

- The dark side of occupation contributes to the continually evolving theory of every aspect of occupation, as people's occupations, their forms, functions, meanings, and contexts, are ever-changing.
- The dark side of occupation is in all practice settings.
- The prevalence of the dark side of occupation in people's lives is a varying yet unknown phenomenon.
- The dark side of occupation can be genuinely threatening to people's health and their lives.

As a closing recommendation, we refer back to Chapter 1, in which Rebecca made a statement for us to contemplate and to respond to:

> Alongside the need for this evolution are many other needs, such as for occupational scientists and occupational therapists to become socially responsible, to act on climate change, to challenge barriers in health, care, and education (such as culture, access, availability, and language) and the ever-increasing political tensions, to promote and advance equality, diversity, human and occupational rights, to strengthen as a global and diverse community, to be proud, to be resilient, to accept when change may be needed, to flourish, and to be kind in a world where there is much unkindness.

References

Biermann, S. (2011). Knowledge, power and decolonization: Implication for non-indigenous scholars, researchers and educators. In G.J.S. Dei (Ed.), *Indigenous philosophies and critical education: A reader* (pp. 386–398). New York: Peter Lang.

Bury, M. (1982). Chronic illness as biographical disruption. *Sociology of Health and Illness*, 4(2), pp. 167–182. doi:10.1111/1467-9566.ep11339939.

Eyres, P., Bannigan, K., & Letherby, G. (2019). An understanding of religious doing: A Photovoice study. *Religions*, 10(4), p. 269. https://doi.org/10.3390/rel10040269.

Froehlich, J. (1992). Occupational therapy interventions with survivors of sexual abuse. *Occupational Therapy in Health Care*, 8(1/2), pp. 1–25. doi:10.1080/J003v08n02_01.

Hammell, K.R. (2017). Critical reflections on occupational justice: Toward a rights-based approach to occupational opportunities. *Canadian Journal of Occupational Therapy*, 84(1), pp. 47–57. doi:10.1177/0008417416654501.

Hammell, K.W., & Iwama, M.K. (2012). Well-being and occupational rights: An imperative for critical occupational therapy. *Scandinavian Journal of Occupational Therapy*, 19(5), pp. 385–394. doi:10.3109/11038128.2011.611821.

Jacobs, K., & MacRae, N. (Eds.) (2017). *Occupational therapy essentials for clinical competence* (3rd ed.). Thorofare, NJ: Slack.

Krishan, A. (2009). What are academic disciplines? Some observations on the disciplinarity vs. interdisciplinarity debate. Retrieved from http://eprints.ncrm.ac.uk/783/1/what_are_academic_disciplines.pdf.

Magalhães, L., Farias, L., Rivas-Quarneti, N., Alvarez, L., & Serrata Malfitano, A.P. (2019). The development of occupational science outside the Anglophone sphere: Enacting global collaboration. *Journal of Occupational Science, 26*(2), pp. 181–192. doi:10.1080/14427591.2018.1530133.

Royal College of Occupational Therapists (2019). About occupational therapy: What is occupational therapy? Retrieved from www.rcot.co.uk/about-occupational-therapy/what-is-occupational-therapy.

Shih, C.H. (2009). Academic colonialism and the struggle for Indigenous knowledge systems in Taiwan. *Social Alternatives, 29*(1), pp. 44–47. Retrieved from http://faculty.ndhu.edu.tw/~cfshih/journal-articles/201003-1.pdf.

Twinley, R. (2013). The dark side of occupation: A concept for consideration. *Australian Occupational Therapy Journal, 60*(4), pp. 301–303. https://doi.org/10.1111/1440-1630.12026.

Twinley, R. (2016). The perceived impacts of woman-to-woman rape and sexual assault, and the subsequent experience of disclosure, reaction, and support on victim/survivors' subjective experience of occupation (Doctoral dissertation, University of Plymouth, UK). Retrieved from https://pearl.plymouth.ac.uk/handle/10026.1/6551

Whalley Hammell, K. (2019). Building globally relevant occupational therapy from the strength of our diversity. *World Federation of Occupational Therapists Bulletin, 75*(1), pp. 13–26. doi:10.1080/14473828.2018.1529480.

Index

Page numbers in **bold** denote tables.

Printed in the United States
By Bookmasters